DR. SEARS'
High-Speed
in 7 Fat Loss
Easy Steps

Al Sears MD, CCN

Published by:

Al Sears, MD • 12794 Forest Hill Blvd., Suite 16 • Wellington, FL 33414
www.alsearsmd.com

Warning-Disclaimer: Dr. Al Sears wrote this book to provide information in regard to the subject matter covered. Every effort has been made to make this book as complete and accurate as possible. The purpose of this book is to educate. The author and the publisher shall have neither liability nor responsibility to any person or entity with respect to any loss, damage, or injury caused or alleged to be caused directly or indirectly by the information contained in this book. The information presented herein is in no way intended as a substitute for medical counseling or medical attention.

Table of Contents

About the Author

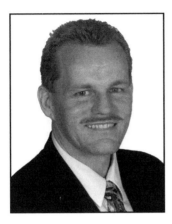

Al Sears, MD continues to see patients at his integrative clinic and research center in Florida where he has developed novel exercise and nutritional systems transforming the lives of over 20,000 patients.

His original contributions and commanding knowledge of alternative medicine have put him at the forefront of anti-aging medicine, both as a lecturer and published author.

Dr. Sears' latest release, ***Your Best Health Under the Sun*...** exposes one of the biggest myths of our time... the misconception that the sun is your enemy. It shows you that sun exposure produces one of the most potent health-boosting substances in your body.

He has written over 500 articles and 6 books in the fields of alternative medicine, anti-aging and nutritional supplementation. He enjoys a worldwide readership and has appeared on over 50 national radio programs, ABC News, CNN and ESPN.

His fifth book, ***PACE: Rediscover Your Native Fitness*** sparked a revolution in the fitness world. An effective alternative to traditional cardio, PACE is practiced worldwide, delivering reliable fat loss an prevention against heart attack and stroke.

In 2005, Dr. Sears' ***12 Secrets to Virility*** shed light on the huge environmental and nutritional problems with virility in our modern world. It gave men a step-by-step guide for maintaining health, strength and masculinity as they age, and became a bestseller during its first month of release.

His third book, ***The Doctor's Heart Cure***, exposed the real causes of the modern epidemic of heart disease with practical how-to advice for building real heart strength and resistance to disease without drugs. It is available in 9 languages and remains a best-seller 4 years after its publication.

In 2000, Dr. Sears' launched his successful ***The T-Factor King of Hormones***. Finally, men were able to take a serious look at virility and discover ways to naturally boost their testosterone.

His first publication, ***21st Century Men's Guide to Prostate Health***, gave men real answers for reducing their risk for common prostate problems long before the problem's exposure with mainstream medicine and the media.

Dr. Sears also publishes a monthly newsletter – Health Confidential – addressing the issues of aging, nutrition and sexual health for men and women and a weekly e-letter called Doctor's House Call.

He is board certified as a clinical nutrition specialist and was appointed to the international panel of experts at **Health Sciences Institute**, (HSI) a worldwide information service for alternative nutritional therapies.

Dr. Sears is a member of the American Academy of Anti-Aging Medicine and is Board Certified in Anti-Aging Medicine. As a pioneer in this new field of medicine, he is an avid researcher and sought after lecturer to thousands of doctors and health enthusiasts.

He is a member of the American College of Sports Medicine and the National Youth Sports Coaches Association. As well as being a sports and fitness coach and a lifelong advocate of exercise programs, Dr. Sears is an ACE certified fitness trainer.

Chapter 1

Discard These 3 Big Fat Lies

Fat Lie #1: You are Genetically Programmed to Get Fat

Many have claimed that getting fat is a consequence of our own success because we are programmed to overeat as a survival strategy. They say that we are only now capable of eating as much as we want, so our predestined genes doom us to either get obese or feel starved.

I want you to just think about this theory for a moment. Are we really designed with such a flaw? What if one clan developed a better spear point and had more success in the hunt? Their own success would cause them to get so fat that they would be unable to defend themselves from a less successful, lean neighboring clan. This kind of genetic predisposition can't survive the rigors of competition for long.

The cause of our modern epidemic of obesity can't be genetic because it is rapidly changing. Genes can't change that fast. It has been caused by recent and rapid changes to our environment.

With dazzling speed in evolutionary terms, we did something completely new with our food. We turned over control of what we eat to someone other than ourselves. Yes, you still decide what you put in your mouth. But our modern food system does not allow you to control its production. This seemingly harmless step toward efficiency has created a big, unexpected (and for most a still unappreciated) problem.

The food producer has an incentive to change what the food consumer eats. Food producers (like producers of anything else) strive for higher profits. Since anyone can acquire and sell our native foods, competition keeps margins slim on traditional foods. But if a food producer makes a new food that doesn't occur in nature, he has created an exclusive product that is, at least for a time, without identical competitors and can demand higher margins.

Rewards in this system can be huge. Five cents worth of wheat and corn syrup are transformed into a three dollar box of cereal. But even man-made products can be copied. So if you have succeeded in convincing a lot of people to eat your unnatural product, copycatters will soon begin whittling away at your enviable margins. In addition to creating an astounding efficiency in man-made food production, this system also creates an incentive to constantly change and keep changing what we eat.

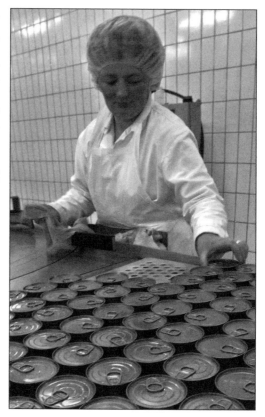

The more unnatural a food's processing, the longer it will preserve a proprietary advantage. Competitors will soon learn a procedure for flaking wheat or puffing rice, but if it uses complicated processing or expensive equipment like "double ion exchange columns" or "ultra-high speed centrifugation", it will hang on to exclusivity and thus higher profits for longer. So the most unnatural foods sustain the highest profits.

Yet there's a fly in the synthetic soup. For this all to work, the food producer must convince you, the food consumer, that his exclusive new food is somehow better than your old nonproprietary native food. Here the process becomes less of a testament to American ingenuity.

Dig below the surface of that package of substitute food and you uncover a monumentally huge and troubling web of corruption and conspiracy to misinform. Yet unlike the exposure and civil punishment of the tobacco industry, the commercial food producers' processing and branding artificial foods as natural, wholesome, and healthy has won the day.

The disengagement and ignorance of medicine over nutrition and the corrupting influence of the world's most powerful political action committees and self-serving government bureaucracies have succeeded in confusing and distorting the truth. By doing so, they were successful in separating you from your last contact with normal eating.

The result has been that the more processed and further from your native food a product is the cheaper it will likely be, the more likely our government will tout it and the more paid "medical research" will appear to support its "health benefits."

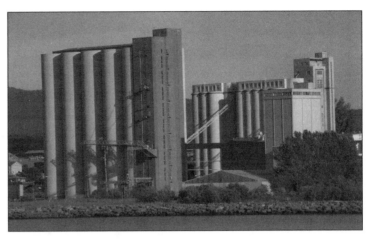

Or put another way, the cheaper, more flavored, more widely available, more advertised, and more supported a food is, the more unnatural to you it really is. So this is why I say you are dieting. Without your awareness you are very likely dieting now. You were born dieting.

Why should you care? Because, currently, there is no better tool to assess a food's healthiness than the exact opposite of all of this. That is, whether it is native to your diet. Theories of nutrition have been unreliable. As you will see, many have come and gone. All nutritional analyses aside, your most reliable guide is still what we have eaten for thousands of years.

A first step toward reversing the modern epidemic of obesity is to simply reverse, as best you can, the recent changes to your diet. This book will help reconnect you with your native eating.

Fat Lie #2: Counting Calories Is the Best Way to Lose Fat

Doctors and nutritionists would have you believe that counting calories is the best way to lose fat. How many times have you heard this misguided advice?

- Calories in, calories out… that's all you need to worry about.
- If you consume more calories than you burn, the rest turns to fat.

• The best way to burn calories is aerobic exercise.

There's only one problem. Applying this theory in practice doesn't usually work.

Your body is not a machine. It's a living, sentient being that has its own "intelligence." It decides on its own how to use the calories you consume. There is no proof that excess calories automatically turn to fat.

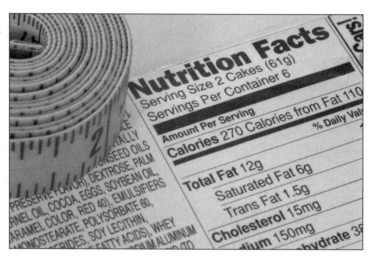

Of course, some people just eat way too much. If you're trying to lose fat but live on fast food, such over consumption will obviously get in your way. But for most people trying to lose weight that's not the problem. And for the majority of people, I tell them: "If you want to lose fat and keep it off, forget about calories."

You may be surprised to hear that. It may sound like a contradiction. Let me explain why I don't believe counting calories is necessary or even very helpful in losing fat. I will tell you in the same way I learned – from a patient's story.

The point is one I was slow to learn. I had to be beaten over the head with it for years before it sunk in.

Dropping Calories Only to Gain More Weight...

A young woman came to my clinic about 12 years ago. We'll call her LS. She was 5 foot 2 and weighed 170 pounds. She had been trying to lose weight for two years but said, *"No matter how little I eat, my weight just keeps going up."*

When I asked her about exercise, she insisted, *"I work as a waitress and I'm on the run for 10 hours a day. And I'm up to working out for 90 minutes 5 times a week."*

I told her to cut her calories to 1600 and see me in two weeks. She did this diligently and brought me a complete record. Her weight went up by four pounds. I told her to bring down her calories to 1400 per day. The result? She gained four more pounds.

I cut her to 1200 then 1000, calories and again she gained weight. Now she lacked energy, couldn't make herself go to the gym anymore, and was feeling depressed.

She still wanted to lose weight. So… I told her to cut her calories to 800 and see me again in two weeks. I never saw her again, and she didn't return the calls from my office. If I could, I would apologize to her and tell her what we did wrong.

The Wrong Strategy for Weight Loss

You have probably heard that conventional diets don't work. History has shown that five out of six people who try to lose weight fail. And more than 90% of those who do succeed in losing weight gain all the weight back within two years.

When you consider the flawed strategy these diets use, this is no surprise. You can't achieve and maintain your ideal weight by starving yourself thin. Even if you could, it would be bad for your health.

Losing weight has been so hard because you've had the wrong tool for the job. If you drop your calories too low and go hungry – forcing your body to lose weight – your body will fight you in this effort. Like I said, your body has a built in "intelligence."

It reacts as if you are starving and will do everything it can to preserve your fat. And when you lose weight through starving yourself, you lose important muscle, bone, fluids and even vital organ mass.

Your body has mechanisms for setting your weight at where it wants it to be. It is similar to the way you set your house temperature with your thermostat.

So the right tool for the job is one that changes your set point. The good news is that you can change these controls through diet and exercise. But they're not the diet and exercise that we used to think. They involve eating differently – not eating less.

5,000 Calories a Day and Still Losing Weight...

At about the same time, I was becoming more perplexed over why my patients were not responding to a low-calorie diet. Then I encountered a patient at the opposite extreme. We'll call him ST.

ST also weighed 170 pounds, the same as LS, the young lady who couldn't burn fat from a low-calorie diet. But ST wanted to **gain** weight.

His trainer had told him to eat as much protein as possible. But he hadn't gained a pound. When this didn't work, he added more protein. He kept adding more protein until he came to see me. Frustrated, he said, *"Doc I'm up to eating like a pig six times a day. I'm stuffed all the time and I can't gain a pound."*

When I looked at his food log, I could hardly believe it. He ate a dozen egg whites a day. He ate 24 ounces of steak at a time, sometimes twice a day. He drank a 40-ounce protein shake twice a day. And in between meals, he would scarf down 36 ounces of canned tuna and pure protein snacks.

When I totaled the calories, he ate between 4500 and 5000 calories a day for the previous 12 weeks. **And he lost six pounds.**

I thought exercise might explain it. But he said, *"No Doc, I'm doing very little. I go to the gym three times a week, but I don't do cardio and I'm out of there in 20 minutes. I don't want to burn the calories..."*

At first, I thought it must be the difference in the rate these two individuals burn calories at rest. This is called the basal metabolic rate (BMR). But to account for such a dramatic difference, the BMR would have to vary by more than 500%.

But research shows only a marginal variation in a person's BMR, which is nowhere near that magnitude. Clearly, something else was in play...

What ST had done was discover by accident the most important principal of healthy weight loss. To make weight loss relatively easy and healthy you must overconsume protein.

I mean you must eat more protein than your body is going to use. Why do this? Because this is what throws the metabolic switch. It tells your body that times are good. When times are good, it doesn't need the stored fat. <u>It can now burn that fat for other things</u>.

In Step One of your *7 Easy Steps*, I'll tell you exactly how much protein you need for high-speed fat loss. First, there's another fat-loss myth that needs to be put down...

Fat Lie #3: Eating Fat Makes You Fat

For 30 years, the American Heart Association, the modern food industry and the media have been telling you the secret to fat loss is a low-fat diet. This is a dangerous mistake.

For years, a handful of us in medicine have been telling you the opposite – that dietary fat is not the problem. And when you eat low fat, you inevitably eat more carbohydrate and inadvertently sacrifice the most important nutrient, protein. This is a prescription for losing vital muscle and turning your body into flab.

All along, we've had a growing body of medical studies backing up our claims. But the governmental organizations have stubbornly clung to their low-fat hypothesis and the media has failed to recognize the mounting evidence against it. But over the last few years, that's started to change...

In 2003, *The New York Times Sunday Magazine* ran a cover story entitled "What If It's All Been a Big Fat Lie?" The article said the American medical establishment's worst nightmare had come true – not only had they been wrong about what constitutes a healthy diet, but their recommendations had made the problem worse... and their critics had been right all along.

Let's be clear... eating a low-fat, high-carb diet not only makes you fatter, but also puts you at risk for a slew of medical problems – from the onset of diabetes to heart disease and stroke.

Enjoy the Food You were Born to Eat...

The *New York Times Magazine* article was largely correct. Hundreds of medical studies have shown that the low-fat, high-starch diet advocated by so many has made Americans fatter and sicker.

An alarming report out of Stockholm University that was released through Sweden's National Food Administration in April found cancer-causing agents in breads, rice, potatoes, and cereals. Starch transforms into a compound called acrylamide when heated. Acrylamide is recognized as a carcinogen by the U.S. Environmental Protection Agency.[1]

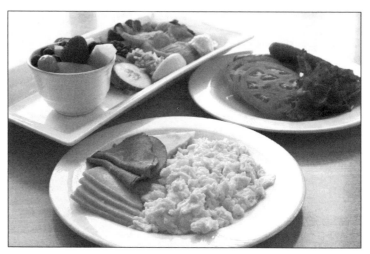

If you want to burn fat, you have to forget about tofu burgers and whole-grain breads. The good news is you can start eating the foods you like. You can eat the things your father probably told you would "put hair on your chest" decades ago – like steak and eggs!

In fact, the *Journal of Nutrition* published a German study that proved the importance of protein. The researchers found that high protein diets boost antioxidant levels. The higher the protein consumed, the higher the antioxidant levels became. Low protein consumption actually seemed to induce the oxidative affects of free radicals.[2]

I've helped hundreds of my own patients use this approach. I've seen them make the transformation from fat and sickly to lean and healthy. My clinic is full of patients who used to take multiple medications and now take none. Along with becoming lean, these men and women see their cholesterols and triglycerides drop, their high blood pressures resolve, their pain of arthritis gone, and their diabetes reversed.

One of the most recent studies has proven that the incorporation of lean meat into the diet helps reduce cholesterol levels. By the way, it didn't matter whether it was white meat or red meat. Both lowered bad LDL cholesterol and raised good HDL cholesterol.[3]

There have also been studies that prove that low-carbohydrate diets improve diabetes. One important study analyzed diabetic patients for eight weeks. Some of the patients ate a diet with 55% of calories from carbohydrates (very similar to the average American's diet). The other group ate a diet where 25% of the calories came from carbohydrates. The group eating the 25% diet experienced a drop in blood sugar levels. People eating the 55% diet experienced a rise in blood sugar levels. Those eating more carbohydrates worsened their diabetic condition.[4]

Our Wellness Research Foundation has also collected compelling scientific evidence that not only the modern epidemic of obesity but many "modern" diseases are either caused or worsened by following the diet that you've been told was healthy.

There is still much to be learned about nutrition. But one thing is becoming increasingly clear. The best diet is the diet that we instinctively want to eat. It's the diet we *were* eating – without the help of modern medicine – for eons.

What Did Your Ancient Ancestors Really Eat?

The earliest evidence of the diet of early man comes from fossils. The record is clear. Early man preferred animal flesh. His whole culture was built around acquiring and consuming meat.

And we can go even further back in time. Man's closest living relative, the chimpanzee, regularly hunts down and consumes animal flesh. The meat is very highly prized with the highest-ranking members consuming their fill first. They show a preference for the fat and the organs of their prey.

When all those vegetarian books were so popular back in the 60s and 70s, primatologists believed most other primates were vegetarians. This was cited as a reason for people to swear off beef and eat bean sprouts instead. I still see this claim being made, but we now know it to be false. Most other primates regularly eat insects, forage for small animals, and routinely hunt down and eat any game they can kill.

Perhaps even more convincing is the data from indigenous cultures. Many of these cultures survived unaffected by the modern world into the 20th century. Anthropologists studied and recorded their dietary habits.

Of particular note is the work of Dr. Weston Price. He traveled throughout the world meticulously documenting their lifestyles. He studied 14 remaining hunter-gatherer cultures.

He discovered two very remarkable features in every culture. One, they were universally lean and lacked the modern constellation of diseases. Two, they all prized and ate meat. There was not a single vegetarian culture.

An extensive study of the health of native people was conducted by Dr. Loren Cordain. Dr. Cordain is an expert on primitive dietary habits and a professor of exercise physiology at Colorado State University. He examined the diets of 229 of the world's remaining native societies. Here's a summary of his findings.

- He also found no vegetarian cultures.
- Game was their principal source of protein and fat.
- Hunted game or fish was highly valued.
- Organ meat was most coveted, often reserved for the privileged.

Dr. Cordain also found hunter-gatherers relied on animal products as their main food source. Animal foods make up 50-65% of the societies' diets. Cordain concluded:

"... this high reliance on animal-based foods coupled with the relatively low carbohydrate content of wild plant foods produces universally characteristic macronutrient consumption ratios in which protein intakes are greater at the expense of carbohydrate." [5]

Ancient vs. Modern Western Diet

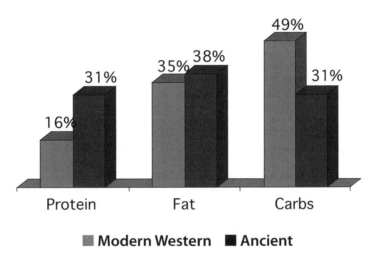

The fact that native pre-agricultural societies universally ate more protein than the average modern diet surprises my patients. <u>They have read that we eat too much protein.</u>

The evidence when taken together makes one conclusion undeniable. A low-fat vegetarian diet has never been the natural diet of man. The truth is the exact opposite. For millions of years man has eaten meat. What's more, meat was universally prized in every primitive culture.

Natives Who Ate Meat Were Never Fat

Politically correct or not, the more meat an indigenous society ate, the healthier it appeared. For instance, the Masai of east Africa, who live on raw milk, cattle meat and blood and organ meat appeared to completely lack dental cavities, obesity, or heart disease.

Among the healthiest of all native groups studied are the Dinkas. They live along the banks of the Nile River and live mostly on fish and shellfish. One western physician who lived among them reported to have never seen a single case of obesity, heart disease, or cancer in 15 years.

The Dawn of High Carb Diets

Ten thousand years ago, people began to domesticate plants and animals. There was a gradual switch from hunting and gathering to farming. Farming could support a larger population. Quality was traded for quantity. This was the start of the Agricultural Revolution.

Archaeologists can identify the Agricultural Revolution in the fossil record. Human remains tell the tale. But not in the way you might think. Skeletal relics can show the age, gender, height, weight, illnesses, and the state of health of an individual. Archaeologists have found that farming communities were more malnourished and disease ridden than their hunter-gatherer predecessors.

Hunter-gatherer skeletons in Greece show that the average height was about 5'9" until the advent of agriculture; then Greeks suddenly shrank to a mere 5'. Even today, the Greek population has not fully regained the height of their primitive predecessors.

The record of native people in the Illinois and Ohio River Valleys also demonstrate the health consequences of agriculture.

"Archaeologists have excavated some 800 skeletons that paint a picture of the health changes that occurred when a hunter-gatherer culture gave way to the intensive maize farming around A. D. 1150 ... these early farmers paid a price for their new-found livelihood. Compared to the hunter-gatherers who preceeded them, the farmers had a nearly 50% increase ... in malnutrition, a fourfold increase in iron-deficiency anemia ...[and] a threefold rise in infectious disease." [6]

Farmers always grow high-carbohydrate crops. There are no other crops. Even the soybean often touted for its high protein is still over 80% carbohydrate. Other staple crops like potatoes, corn, wheat, and rice are all over 90% carbohydrate.

Farming communities no longer receive the range of nutrients that hunter-gatherers had. And, farmers do not consume high amounts of protein. Malnourished farmers were more susceptible to disease.

The record is consistent. When hunter-gatherers switched to farming, their fat and protein intake went down and their carbohydrate intake went up. The incidence of malnutrition and diseases rose in every case I can find.

Of course, the sudden rise in the modern constellation of diseases did not go unnoticed. In the middle of the last century, it began to be identified as the modern plague.

Fat is Wrongly Blamed for Making People Fat and Diseased

You can blame a reductionist view of health; you can blame the commercial interest of food producers or slick Madison Avenue marketing, but for one reason or another, the cause of the problem was misread.

<u>Without real evidence, fat was identified as the culprit</u>. It was not known that native diets included more fat than modern diets. Endocrinology or the study of hormones was not considered.

If we can divorce ourselves from the prejudice about fat, the endocrinology is really quite simple. Your body controls fat building. Hormones are used to set the controls. The hormone insulin controls fat.

How much insulin do you secrete in response to a fat laden meal? Zero. Insulin is secreted in response to carbohydrate. Eat more carbohydrate and you will secrete more insulin and build more fat, all other things being equal. Fat in the diet, in contrast, is neutral.

Scientists have even recently identified the cellular machinery that turns carbohydrates into fat. Researchers at the University of Texas Southwestern

Medical Center found a protein in cells called ChREBP. It converts excess dietary carbohydrates into fat stores.

Americans Abandon Fat and Go Carb Crazy

In 1977, George McGovern led a Senate committee that released its "Dietary Goals for the United States." The publication advised that Americans drastically cut their dietary fat intake. And, according to the "Dietary Goals," fat was the cause of illnesses sweeping the nation.

The National Institute of Health jumped on the "ban fat" wagon. In 1984, NIH announced that Americans must cut their fat intake. In response, the food industry quickly produced a slew of "low-fat" products. But without the tasty fat, the food produced was bland. High amounts of sugar became a common additive.

Americans replaced fat with refined carbohydrates and sugar. The amount of calories from fat in the American diet decreased. And, the amount of calories from refined carbohydrates increased … dramatically.

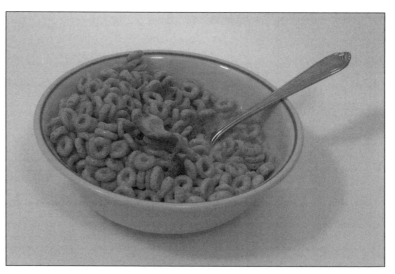

Cereals were cheap to produce and could be sold at a huge profit. When Kellogg and other early proponents of cereals started their health farms, they preached that modern society was oversexed. Eating cereal, they claimed, would solve the problem.

As bizarre as this and the other inflated and unsubstantiated claims were, there might be a twisted kernel of truth. Cholesterol is the building block for testosterone. If you deprive yourself of animal fat, your testosterone will go down.

Testosterone deficiency has the worst kinds of consequences for men (impotence, depression, obesity, and fatigue to name a few). I've seen evidence for this firsthand. Some of the most severe testosterone deficiencies I've encountered were in men eating a very low-fat diet. Often, they had gotten this advice from their physicians.

Your Body Needs Essential Fats

The main problem I have with low fat is that it also means high carb. Excessive intake of carbohydrate is the central dietary problem in my patient population. But there is another problem emerging from the low-fat advice. The lower fat intake itself can be detrimental to your health.

One study published in the *Journal of Clinical Nutrition* found that low-fat diets affect calcium absorption. The study found low-fat diets were associated with 20% lower calcium absorption than higher-fat diets.[7]

The State University of New York at Buffalo also found that low-fat diets cause health problems. The researchers found that people who eat low-fat diets develop weaker immune systems.[8]

A certain amount of fat is critical to absorb vitamins. The fat-soluble nutrients like vitamins A, D, E, and K and CoQ10 cannot be absorbed without fat.

Ditch the Diets and Return Your Native Fitness

The good news is that fixing this mess is not as hard as you might think. What was caused by 10 millennia of farming and worsened by weak science and bad advice can be fixed by you alone.

Follow a few simple rules for selecting your food. You will find a guide to selecting healthy "real natural" foods in this book. You will be able to eat better-tasting foods and feel more satisfied.

And don't be worried that eating meat is going to drive up your cholesterol.

Now you've just learned why you shouldn't believe the low-fat diet lie.

In the next chapter we'll look at how years of misguided diet advice has lead to an unhealthy obsession with carbs.

References:

1 Swedish Scientists Find Cancer Agent in Staple Foods Reuters News: April 23, 2002

2 Journal of Nutrition 2000; 130: 2889-2896

3 Journal of the American College of Nutrition 2000; 19(3): 351-360

4 Journal of American College of Nutrition 1998; 17: 595-600

5 Cordain L, et al., Plant-animal subsistence ratios and macronutrient energy estimations in worldwide hunter-gatherer diets. Am J Clin Nutr March 2000: 71(3); 682-692

6 Diamond J The Worst Mistake in the Human Race. Discover Magazine May 1987 p. 65

7 American Journal of Clinical Nutrition Aug 2000; 72: 466-471

8 Medicine Science of Sports Exercise July 2000; 32(7): 389-95

Chapter 2

Kick These New Foods to the Curb

Don't Fall for These "New Foods"

You often hear that fast food is bad for you because it's too high in fat. Fast food can be bad for you all right. But not for the reasons you might think. Ancient man averaged 38% of their calories from fat. The typical American consumes 35% of their calories from fat. <u>We are eating less fat than our ancestors.</u>

In this chapter, I'll explain the real pitfalls of fast food so you can make smarter choices for a quick lunch. I'll also reveal why diets and "health foods" often steer you in the wrong direction.

Carbs: The Real Culprit Behind Obesity

Processed carbohydrates are the real major cause of obesity and heart disease in the modern diet. Government health agencies giving you that bad "low-fat" health advice completely ignore this fact: When you choose your food solely by the quantity of fat it contains you will inevitably consume more carbohydrates. And, the typical lower-fat fast food choices are loaded with the worst kinds of processed carbs. They are in very high quantities in:

- Breaded and fried fish and chicken
- Oversized white-flour buns
- French fried potatoes
- Sugar-based sodas

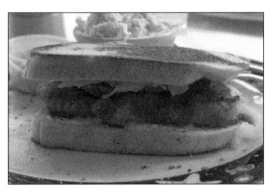

The media has perpetuated the myth that animal fat is responsible for the weight gain and high cholesterol levels

---

associated with modern living. Low fat may be the most profitable food but its recommended consumption is based on a false assumption.

The fact is that animal fat has been a central part of our diet for millions of years. During this period, both obesity and heart disease were rare phenomena. Processed carbohydrates were not a part of that diet. Excessive amounts of these unnatural carbs combined with excessive calories made us fat with soaring cholesterols, **not** the quantity of fat.[1]

Many studies have shown that low-carb diets are more effective than low-fat diets for reversing our overweight condition. The most recent study reported in the *Journal of Family Practice* concluded, "Low carbohydrate diets result in more weight loss than low-fat/low-calorie diets after six months, with no adverse impact on lipids, bone density, or blood pressure." [2]

All Fats Are Not Created Equal...

You don't have to avoid fat just because it's fat. But, not all fats are equal. The quality of fat in fast food meat is indeed among some of the poorest you can eat. But it has more to do with the environment of the meat than whether it's red meat or white.

The proportion of unhealthy omega-6 fats to healthy omega-3 fats has changed from a ratio of 2 to 1 in Paleolithic times to 20 to 1 today. The meat is also adulterated and polluted today compared to the meat our ancestors hunted. This is why I recommend buying grass-fed beef or wild game. Grass-fed meat has six times more omega-3s than grain-fed meat.[3]

What about the fast food fish? Fish does have the heart healthy omega-3 fats. However, the health benefit of fish is dependent upon how it is prepared. A recent study published in *Circulation* followed 4,000 participants for nine years. Researchers found that those who ate fried fish failed to reap any of the heart protection benefit normally associated with fish consumption.[4]

And, there are other problems with eating the fried fish or chicken sandwiches. Let's go back to the fish sandwich and cheeseburger comparison again.

The McDonald's Sandwich Test

Menu Item	Total Fat	Carbohydrates	Protein	Calories
Fish Sandwich	26 g	45 g	15 g	470
Chicken Sandwich	26 g	46 g	22 g	500
Cheeseburger	14 g	35 g	15 g	330

Notice that the only thing the fish doesn't have more of is the most vital macronutrient for good health – protein. The cheeseburger and the fish both have 15 g of protein. The biggest difference is that the fish and chicken have more processed carbs. These extra calories, fat, and carbs are not natural to fish but are products of McDonald's processing. Additionally, the frying of fish and chicken in vegetable oils with trans fats creates an even bigger health problem.

Man-Made Fats Directly Linked to Heart Disease

A couple of decades ago, food manufacturers discovered that a process called hydrogenation could transform liquid vegetable oils into solids. This allowed cheap corn and soy substitutes for animal fats like lard and butter. They also vastly increased the shelf-lives over their natural counterparts', further increasing profits. Since these transformed oils do not exist in nature, their use in our food was an untested experiment. An experiment conducted on a huge scale on an uninformed public.

We are only now beginning to register the results of this experimental deviance from the historical norm of dependence on natural fats. It turns out that the hydrogenation process produces trans fatty acids in the oil. Trans fatty acids have now been shown not to decrease risk of heart disease at all. In fact they increase your risk of heart disease. Even worse, they interfere with the processing of the healthy fats your body needs. And, they may cause cancer.

Today our diet is full of trans fatty acids. They are in those packaged pastries that have become so ubiquitous. They are in our margarine and our bread. They are even in the Oreo cookies we feed our children. And, Mc-

Donald's and other fast food chains add them into their French fries during the cooking. They are the very cheapest oils, and McDonald's claims they improve the flavor of their fries.

In 2001, *Lancet* published a comprehensive Dutch study addressing the effects of consuming *trans* fatty acid. Researchers found that trans fatty acid intake was directly associated with **increased risk** of coronary heart disease.[5]

In July 2003, the FDA declared that Nutrition Facts labels must list *trans* fats. Since then, many fast food chains are promising to either reduce or eliminate the use of trans fats. As of this writing, McDonald's is testing new trans-fat-free oils for their French fries but has yet to introduce them to their restaurants.

"Health Foods" that Make You Sick

You'll see plenty of packaged foods labeled natural and healthy. Fact is, real health food doesn't come in packages. Let's take a closer look.

- You buy energy bars for extra energy while filling your nutritional needs on the fly.

Fact: These bars contain hydrogenated vegetable oils and trans fats that rob you of vital nutrients, create fatigue, and promote heart disease.

- You buy sports drinks that promise nutrients to give you a competitive edge.

Fact: These drinks contain high-fructose corn syrup that induces a hormonal reaction that blocks important minerals, compromising your performance.

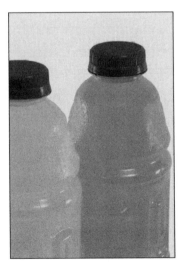

- You buy low-fat foods believing the claims that they'll help you lose weight.

Fact: Low-fat foods contain artificial sweeteners that create cravings, lead to further weight gain and produce formaldehyde – toxic to your liver and brain.

Food manufacturers have the gall to promote these foods as "healthy." Most Americans are unaware of the scientific studies linking these adulterated foods to heart disease, diabetes, and cancer.

Artificial Sweeteners Can Poison

Manufacturers developed a chemical process to produce high-fructose corn syrup (HFCS) about 25 years ago. They prefer it to more natural sweeteners because it's cheaper than dirt, spoil resistant, super-sweet, and easy to mix and store. Today Americans consume more HFCS than old-fashioned sugar.[6] You'll even find HFCS in most supposed health foods such as sports drinks, fruit juice drinks, energy bars, cereals, and yogurt.

Research shows that fructose promotes disease more than other sugars. For example, every cell in your body metabolizes glucose but only the liver metabolizes fructose. Animals fed high-fructose diets develop fatty liver deposits and cirrhosis, similar to the livers of alcoholics.

A study conducted by Dr. Lee Gross at Harvard found that the increased use of processed foods with corn syrup directly parallels a dramatic rise in diabetes and obesity.[7]

Fructose interferes with the absorption of copper. Researchers at the USDA found that the combination of low copper and high fructose could lead to serious heart problems. Rats with normal life spans of two years died after just five weeks from heart disease when they ate a diet high in fructose and low in copper. Researchers abruptly stopped a similar human study when four of the twenty-four subjects developed heart abnormalities. High fructose diets also reduce stores of chromium, a mineral essential for normal insulin functioning.[8]

So, you figure you'll switch to the diet version of these "health foods"? Not so fast…

NutraSweet Linked to Disease

Aspartame, known as NutraSweet and Equal, came to the market in 1981. Before it debuted as an artificial sweetener, the U.S. military classified it as a neurotoxin. Now it's in over 5000 products. You'll find it in foods labeled healthy like teas, sports drinks, yogurts, cereals and shake mixes. It's in most of the foods marked "Diet" and "Sugar Free."

Aspartame causes a wide array of problems from memory loss to brain tumors. It is a complex synthetic molecule. Phenylalanine makes 50% and 40% aspartic acid. Aspartic acid eats holes in the brains of laboratory animals.[9]

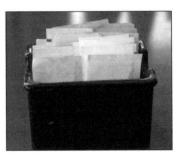

Nutrasweet is commonly in "low-cal" baked products. Dr. Jeffery Bada at the University of California found that when you heat phenylalanine above 85 degrees, it breaks down into toxic methanol, formaldehyde (embalming fluid), formic acid (fire ant venom) and diketopiperazine (DKP).[10]

Just how bad is this? Studies link aspartame to brain tumors, blindness, chronic fatigue, fibromyalgia, Lupus, Alzheimer's, Lou Gehrig's disease, Multiple Sclerosis, Lyme disease, Graves Disease, lymphoma and heart disease among others.[11] I'll give you more surprises about artificial sweeteners in chapter 4.

In the next chapter we will look at how you can avoid common dieting mistakes.

References:

1 Atkins, R., Atkins for Life, St. Martin's Press 2003: 53-54.

2 McCarter, D., Low-carbohydrate diet effective for adults. The Journal of Family Practice, July 2003, Vol 52, NO 7: 515.

3 Robinson, J. Why Grass Fed is Better, Vashon Island Press 2000:12.

4 Mozaffarin D. et al., Cardiac benefits of fish consumption may depend on the type of fish meal consumed. Circulation 2003; 107: 1372-1377

5 Oomen C. at al., Association between trans fatty acid intake and 10-year risk of coronary heart disease in Zutphen Elderly Study. Lancet 2001; 357: 746-751

6 Hallfrisch, Judith, Metabolic Effects of Dietary Fructose, FASEB Journal 4 (June 1990): 2652-2660.

7 American Journal of Clinical Nutrition, November 2002 Vol. 76, No. 5, 911-922.

8 http://www.menstuff.org/issues/byissue/highfructose.html#dangers, The Dangers of Corn Syrup

9 Possible Neuralgic Effects of Aspartame, http://www.dorway.com/wurtman1.html

10 Bada, Jeffrey, "NutraSweet Health and Safety Concerns." Document # Y 4.L11/4:S HR6.100, November 3, 1987, page 456-458.

11 Aspartame Toxicity Information Center, http://www.holisticmed.com/aspartame/

Chapter 3
How to Avoid These Common Dieting Mistakes

Americans are too fat and getting fatter. According to the National Center for Health Statistics, over 60% of Americans are now overweight. Yet we are the biggest dieters with more diets every day. What's going on here?

One interpretation is that our diets are **making** us fatter. At the very least, we have to conclude that the diets are not working. The USDA food pyramid has contributed to the startling rise in obesity over the past decade.

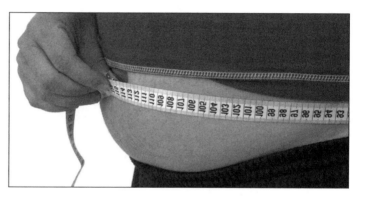

The USDA pyramid recommends a diet based on grain. The base, and largest section, of this pyramid is grain. And it gives less emphasis to proteins and fats. The Harvard pyramid gives even less emphasis to meat. Harvard also recommends eating whole grains with every meal.

Big Problems with the USDA and Harvard Food Pyramids		
Category	USDA Food Pyramid	Harvard Healthy Eating Food Pyramid
Bread, Cereal, Rice, Pasta	Eat 6-11 servings daily	Eat whole grains at every meal
Red meat, fish, poultry, eggs	Eat only 2-3 servings daily	Eat red meat sparingly, eat others 0-2 servings daily

The U.S. Department of Agriculture created the first USDA pyramid in 1992. It may not be a coincidence that it advises us to eat 6 to 11 servings of grain products per day. Nevertheless, this is one of the biggest problems with the pyramid.

Unfortunately, Harvard didn't do much better. The Harvard pyramid meant to solve the problem by advising only *whole*-grains. This switch is healthier for other reasons. But whole grain bread actually spikes blood sugar much the same as white bread.

Nutritionally, grains are almost all starch. They cause a rise in blood sugar. The increased blood sugar then causes a surge of insulin. Over time this increases your risk of diabetes and heart disease. It will also make you fat.

The *International Journal of Obesity* reported a study comparing starches and weight. Subjects who ate a low-starch diet weighed markedly less than those who ate a high-starch diet.[1]

Both pyramids lack healthy protein. Protein is imperative when trying to avoid obesity. New proof has come from the *Journal of Arteriosclerosis, Thrombosis, and Vascular Biology*. They found a mechanism induced by protein. The high-protein diet increased a substance called PAI-1 in the blood. The scientists then showed that PAI-1 inhibits the production of fat.[2]

A "New" Take on a Bad Idea…

Then in 2005, the USDA released a "new" version of their food pyramid. If you haven't seen it, let me save you the trouble. It:

- Has a confusing design with no concrete ideas.

- Gives no hard advice on which foods you should eat.

- Gives no hard advice on which foods you should avoid.

- Completely ignores the primary dietary problem: the over consumption of carbohydrates, particularly sugary processed foods and drinks.

It's clear that once again, the USDA bowed to pressures from the food industry. By not giving any specific information, they didn't offend any particular food maker. They also allow for "discretionary calories," which is their way of avoiding the condemnation of any foods.

That should be expected, considering that 6 of the 11 members of the Dietary Guidelines Advisory Committee have financial ties to the food industry.[3] Not surprisingly, grains once again form the base of the pyramid. To make matters worse, they suggested that 50% of these grains should come from breads, pastas, and breakfast cereals. Which breakfast cereals, I wonder? The all starch ones or the starch plus added sugar ones?

The new food pyramid, just like the old one, will make you fat and increase your risk of disease.

The key should be rebalancing the natural proportions of the three macronutrients: proteins, carbohydrates and fats.

Dr. Sears' Healthy Food Pyramid

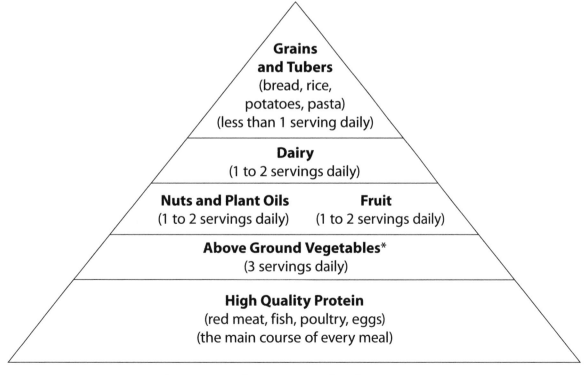

Grains and Tubers
(bread, rice, potatoes, pasta)
(less than 1 serving daily)

Dairy
(1 to 2 servings daily)

Nuts and Plant Oils
(1 to 2 servings daily)

Fruit
(1 to 2 servings daily)

Above Ground Vegetables*
(3 servings daily)

High Quality Protein
(red meat, fish, poultry, eggs)
(the main course of every meal)

Corn is not in this category. I classify it as a grain.

Use the Power of the "Big 3" Nutrients to Burn Fat and Build Muscle

There are three macronutrients: protein, fat, and carbohydrates. Your body deals with each differently. They each induce a different hormonal response independent of the number of calories you eat. Carbohydrates induce insulin secretion and fat building while protein induces growth hormone secretion and muscle building.

Body muscle and body fat both then affect your metabolism. For instance, muscle will stimulate testosterone, masculinization, and energy-burning while fat will stimulate estrogen, feminization, and energy conservation. These responses by your body were not in the old equations but make the critical difference.

Carbohydrates are the unhealthiest foods you can ingest. But the American Medical Association has managed to focus on the one macronutrient that really doesn't matter: fat.

Natural fat is really an inert substance. Fat really doesn't matter. Quality protein is the key to good nutrition. Protein promotes muscle growth and overall health. Protein is chock full of other nutrients that support a healthy body. Carbohydrates make the body insulin resistant. They also provide a home for fat stores.

Dr. Robert C. Atkins understood this. He was a pioneer in the study of macronutrients and their impact on weight gain and loss.

Atkins: What He Got Right… What He Got Wrong…

With his radical low-carb diet, Dr. Robert Atkins dared to confront conventional nutrition. His innovative approach served as a lightning rod. His ensuing persecution exposed the medical profession's closed-minded intolerance of new ideas. And their stubborn misdiagnosis of the real problem with the American diet.

Dr. Atkins' radical view on carbs actually turned out to be right. But he didn't get everything right...

I met Dr. Robert Atkins at a conference here in West Palm Beach on a Sunday in April of 2003. The next day, he returned home to New York City. By the following Tuesday, Dr. Atkins was no more.

He slipped on an icy sidewalk hitting his head. Doctors performed emergency surgery to remove a blood clot from his brain. He fell into a coma during the procedure and died the next day.

Dr. Robert Atkins opened the eyes of the world to a revolutionary vision of nutrition. With his death, the world lost one of the most influential nutritional pioneers of our time. I regret that he will not be around to witness the continued advancement of the diet and health connection that we champion at our *Wellness Research Foundation*.

The Man Who Sparked a Revolution in Nutrition

Atkins first began to research the low-carb approach in the 1960s. He had gained about 30 pounds during medical school and looked for a way to shed the extra weight. Atkins found research about low-carb diets, of all places, in the *Journal of the American Medical Association*. Using their research protocol, he successfully lost the weight, thus sparking over 40 years of low-carb research, practice, and experimentation.

What did Dr. Atkins say that was so different? He made two very contrarian claims.

- One, Americans are fat not because they eat too much fat but because they eat too many carbohydrates.
- Two, the best way to lose weight was not a low-fat diet but a low-carb diet.

Until that time, everyone presumed that weight was determined by a simple relationship of physics: Calories consumed minus calories burned equals weight gain or loss.

Atkins was the first to popularize an alternative. He pointed out that if you take two groups of people and feed them the same number of calories but give one low fat and the other low carb, the low-carb group will lose more weight.

This contradicted what doctors and nutritionists had been telling their patients for decades. The medical mainstream could not (and for the most part still can't) accept this.

But it's a fact. Not only do I agree with Dr. Atkins' diagnosis of the cause of American obesity, but the best science does as well. Independent and accredited research has finally proved what Atkins knew for nearly his entire life. Unfortunately, it has only been in the past couple of years that science has vindicated the low-carb theory.

Mainstream nutritionists still intensely oppose his approach. Old views die hard. But with a mound of scientific evidence, the public view of nutrition is shifting.

The "Big Fat Lie" Exposed

A few years ago, the *New York Times* article, "What If It's All Been a Big Fat Lie" revived the Atkins controversy. The article busted the myth that low-fat diets are healthy.

New research has prompted even the staunchest critics to take notice. In 2004, the mainstream media reported on a landmark study that compared the American Heart Association's low-fat diet to the Atkins' diet. The Atkins' diet produced greater weight loss and lowered cholesterol and triglycerides much more effectively than the low-fat diet.

Atkins was right about the problem. Starches and sugars made Americans fat – not too much dietary fat. But here's where we part: I do not agree with his dietary solution.

Atkins and the Difference between "Good" and "Bad" Fats

Atkins realized that fat doesn't make you fat. But he didn't warn people about the bad fats. An excess of omega-6 fatty acids – the kind you find in grain-fed beef – and man-made trans fatty acids are dangerous and contribute to strokes, heart attacks, and heart disease.

Atkins said any fat is okay. But I don't recommend you eat sausage, hot dogs, cheesecake, and truffles for weight loss or for any other health change. It is true that fat is relatively inert at affecting the hormonal control of your metabolism, but there are other reasons why you do not want to dine on modern western derived fat.

Fat from grain-fed animals is not "natural" fat. It's adulterated by the unnatural living conditions of the animals. The animals are prevented from getting normal exercise and fed a diet of grains instead of grasses.

This makes for an obese and diseased animal. Additionally, all of the herbicides, pesticides, toxins, and hormones that the animal has been exposed to collect in the fat. When you eat this animal fat, you are eating from the cesspool of these animal warehouses.

The vegetable fat that you get in the modern western diet is an abomination. It is not the same as the fat in our natural environment. Vegetable fats are highly processed to extend their shelf lives. The processing creates unhealthy hydrogenation and cancer causing "trans" fatty acids.

Trans-fat is the result of hydrogenation. When a hydrogen molecule is added to vegetable oils, it turns them to fatty solids. These fatty solids replace animal fats, allowing food makers to label their products "cholesterol free."

Industry took away many of the good fats we need – and said they were bad. As a substitute, they gave us man-made fats, which turned out to be dangerous.

Where to find trans-fat:

- Most hardened margarines and shortenings
- Salad dressing and mayonnaise
- Fried fast foods, even those fried in commercial "vegetable oils"
- Corn snacks and chips
- French fries, fried chicken or fish
- Biscuits, rolls, breads, cakes, cookies, crackers and doughnuts

After years of widespread use, numerous studies link trans-fats to heart attacks, strokes, and cancer to name just a few of their many problems. They have proven to increase your LDL (bad) cholesterol. What's worse, they decrease your HDL (good) cholesterol. They also cause inflammation and rob your brain and heart of the real fats you need.[4]

Ironically, doctors recommended these "low-fat" products for years, thinking they were helping their patients. Dr. Walter Willett, Chairman of the Department of Nutrition at the Harvard School of Public Health had this to say:

"There was a lot of resistance from the scientific community because a lot of people had made their careers telling people to eat margarine [containing trans-fats] instead of butter... When I was a physician in the 1980's, that's what I was telling people to do and unfortunately we were often sending them to their graves prematurely." [5]

Clinical Evidence Backs Up Atkins' Low-Carb Approach

There are dozens of clinical studies that back up Atkins' revolutionary approach. Here are just a few:

Nutrition Week reported preliminary results of a study performed by Heritage Medical Center. Researchers looked at the effect of a low-carb diet on participants with metabolic syndrome.

Metabolic syndrome is a diet-induced disease that leads to cholesterol problems, obesity, lack of energy, high blood pressure, and diabetes. Over 100 participants ate a low-carb diet for 18 months. The participants' LDL (bad cholesterol) reduced by an average of 82%. HDL (good cholesterol) scores increased by an average of 30%.

The journal *Obesity Research* published a study that showed the effect of dietary protein on bone loss. Sixty-five subjects participated in a six-month study. Half of the participants ate a high-protein diet, while the other half ate a low-protein diet.

After six months, the group eating high protein lost more weight than the low protein group. Bone mineral loss was markedly higher in the low protein group.

Atkins may be the father of diet trends, but he was certainly not the only one to influence modern diets.

Nine Reasons to Avoid the South Beach Diet

Another popular modern day diet is the South Beach diet. Author, Dr. Agatston gets a few things right including the importance of low-carb foods and that low-fat diets don't work. However, the many flaws with this diet make it dangerous.

Here are nine reasons you should avoid the South Beach Diet.

1. It fails to address the real cause of the American epidemic of obesity. Dr. Agatston completely neglects mentioning how there has been a deviation from natural eating habits and then doesn't offer a way to get back to a natural diet.

2. It fails to give the single best fat-loss tip. Dr. Agatston fails to mention the importance of eating more protein. As you will learn in chapter 5, overconsuming protein programs your body to burn fat.

3. It calls bad carbs "good." While following a low-carb diet is healthy, avoiding them all together is impossible. The carbs you find in vegetables are much better for you than the carbs you find in starchy foods. But Dr. Agatston is mistaken when he says that whole-grain

breads are "good" carbs. This is far from the truth. Bread (whole-grain or white) will make you fat. Not a good idea for weight loss.

4. <u>It is too laid back when it comes to exercise</u>. Exercise is a critical part of weight loss. Dr. Agatston's exercise is all the same approach is misguided. You will learn more about my exercise philosophy in chapter 9.

5. <u>It follows the old myth about saturated fat</u>. Dr. Agatston still believes that saturated fat is the enemy. Some high-quality saturated fat needs to be part of a healthy diet. What really matters is that you get it from the right source. A good source is meat from animals, but it's important to eat grass-fed meat and not grain-fed.

6. <u>It gives dangerous misguidance on the trans-fat issue</u>. Early on Dr. Agatston mentions that trans-fats are dangerous, but later he tells you that French fries and potato chips are healthier choices than a baked potato because of the fat in which they are cooked. Where he got that idea, I'll never know. French fries and potato chips tend to be extremely high in trans-fats and are some of the most unhealthy foods in existence. If you want to lose weight, you won't do it by eating French fries and potato chips.

7. <u>It gives wrong advice about eating fish</u>. Dr. Agatston further shows his lack of dietary knowledge by recommending fish without pointing out the right kind of fish. He fails to mention that it's best to eat wild fish that only comes from a pristine environment such as Alaska. Farm-raised fish, on the other hand, are less nutritious than wild and tend to have high levels of mercury and other toxins.

8. <u>It recommends aspartame</u>. Telling millions of people to use aspartame instead of sugar is reckless. Aspartame is a dangerous neurotoxin linked to many health problems and diseases including seizures, diabetes, and cancer. Once inside your body, aspartame breaks down into poisonous by-products including formaldehyde, also known as embalming fluid.

9. <u>Weight loss is not permanent with this diet</u>. It doesn't teach you the proper way to eat for long-term weight loss. If you start eating natu-

ral, whole foods like our ancestors did for millions of years, weight loss will come easy.

What You Need to Know about other Popular Fad Diets

Here's my take on these other popular fad diets.

Eat to Win: This diet, popularized by tennis pro Martina Navratilova, centers on carbohydrate loading. For the extremely active, initial success does occur. But eventually, excessive carbohydrate intake leads to weight gain – even in athletes. The only time it would be appropriate to eat more than 60% of your calories from carbohydrates is a few days preceding a marathon run or Iron Man triathlon.

The Zone: The Zone diet focuses on the importance of macronutrient ratio. The recommendation is 40% protein, 30% fat, and 30% carbohydrate. The positive aspect of this diet is its emphasis on protein. However, the recommendation of 30% carbohydrate may not be appropriate for all men, especially for those who want to achieve a significant weight loss. The adherence to a fixed ratio is artificial. It is better to change your ratios depending on where you currently are and what your goals are.

Scarsdale: The merit of this diet is its high-protein and low-carb recommendation. Unfortunately, it still adheres to the failed low-fat recommendation. This is likely to lead to nutritional deficiencies. It also interferes with normal satiation of your appetite.

Carb Addict's: This diet centers on the notion of carbohydrate addiction. The reason many people have been successful on this diet is it limits the consumption of carbohydrates to one hour a day at dinnertime.

The major problem with this diet is that it results in higher insulin levels. Not eating adequately to satisfy your hunger, then binging is the perfect way to keep your insulin high. Over time, this can lead to increased risk of heart disease and diabetes.

As a side note, I don't really buy into the modern trend of calling behavioral choices "addictions." The fact is, everything you eat goes into your mouth as a result of a conscious choice.

Sugar Busters: This diet correctly identifies sugar and refined carbohydrates as the major cause of the modern epidemic of obesity and weight gain. It also encourages high protein. But it falls short because of its low-fat, whole-grain advice. Although higher in nutrients than refined carbohydrates, whole grains still boost insulin production.

Protein Power: This diet is based on sound principles. And it works! Beyond the good advice of high protein, low carbohydrate, it stresses the importance of quality protein and fat. It also offers three plans in varying degrees of restriction.

No Grain: This diet accurately portrays grains as the cause of weight gain. It also pays attention to the importance of quality protein like grass-fed beef. What I don't care for about this diet is the same thing that bothers me about the Sugar Addict's diet: the concept of addiction. It gives you the message that you're weak and can't control your own eating habits. That's just not true.

Neanderthin: I like this diet more than any other I have seen published. It centers on the diet of our ancestors. Its basic premise is, "If you couldn't prepare this food on your own, armed with nothing but a sharp stick, don't eat it!"

I think it's one of the healthiest diets you can choose. It focuses on quality protein and fat and complete abstinence from agriculturally produced foods. The only differences I have from this diet are its restriction of beans and dairy.

Beans are a good source of reasonably high-quality protein. You shouldn't rely on them to meet all your protein needs, but I really don't see anything wrong with eating them if you like them and tolerate them well.

In the following table, there is a comparison of these popular diets by amounts of macronutrients and the benefits and problems with each one.

The table describes the amount of macronutrients in each diet as high, normal, or low. These terms correspond with the following percentage values:

High   40% and above
Normal   30-39%
Low   29% and below

Comparison of Macronutrient-Based Diets

Name of Diet	Protein	Fat	Carb	Benefit	Problem
Atkins	High	High	Low	Identifies refined carbs as culprit	Poor quality meat filled with nitrates, toxins, wrong fat
Eat to Win	Low	Low	High	Short-term weight loss for extremely active people	Overconsumption of carbs eventually leads to weight gain
Zone	High	Normal	Normal	High protein consumption. Good fats	The 40-30-30- ratio not ideal for everyone
Scarsdale	High	Low	Low	High protein consumption	Too low in fat. Allows no food substitutions
Carb Addict's	High	Low	Low	Weight loss occurs if dieter strictly follows plan	One hour a day can eat anything (usually high carb)
Sugar Busters	High	Low	Normal	Identifies carbs as culprit. High protein consumption	May be too low in fat to satiate appetite
Protein Power	High	Normal	Low	Focuses on quality protein and quality fat, limits carbs	No major but some see as restrictive
No Grain	Normal	Normal	Low	Identifies grains as culprit. Quality protein	Focuses on the notion of addiction
Neanderthin	High	High	Low	Stresses importance of animal protein and fat	No major. Some may see it as restrictive
South Beach	High	Normal	Normal	Uses higher consumption of lean protein	Encourages whole grain consumption

The Hidden Diet Danger: Sugar Substitutes

Both Atkins and the USDA never talk about the dangers of sweetened food. An excess of regular sugar is bad enough. But artificial sweeteners pose an even bigger threat.

It's been 125 years since the discovery of the first sugar substitute. But attempts to find something sweeter than sugar but without the calories has repeatedly failed.

Far from finding a panacea for our sweet tooth, the industry has launched one product after another with health problems far exceeding those of sugar itself.

In 1879, Johns Hopkins University scientists discovered saccharin by accident.[6] You know saccharin by its brand name Sweet 'N Low. In recent decades, the little pink packets caused a great deal of controversy because they caused bladder cancer in lab rats.

You would have to drink a lot of soda to equal the amount of saccharin given to the rats. However, all products containing saccharin must bear the warning that it may be hazardous to your health.

In 1976 high-fructose corn syrup (HFCS) was introduced. It is the most common sweetener on the market, generating $4.5 billion in annual sales.[7] HFCS is made from cornstarch, fructose, and glucose. But it's a genetically modified product and is completely unnatural.

HFCS sweetens a wide variety of products. It is in soda, Ocean Spray CranApple juice, Gatorade, Campbell's tomato soup, Oreos, Chips Ahoy, Smucker's jellies, Heinz tomato ketchup, Kraft's Thousand Islands salad dressing. It is even found in so-called health foods like Slim Fast meal bars, Arizona Green Tea, SoBe Green Tea, and Kellogg's Raisin Bran.

What's interesting about Arizona Green Tea is that it also contains plum juice. Apparently, the plum juice didn't make it sweet enough so they added HFCS. Why is it in so many food items? Because it is cheaper than natural fruit sweeteners. The syrup is also easier to blend than sucrose.

HFCS is absorbed differently than other sweeteners. This difference may contribute to the obesity problem in America. Fructose produces high levels of insulin and disturbs the flow of two hormones that are critical in appetite control. Leptin is inhibited and ghrelin is stimulated by HFCS which may lead you to overeat and gain weight.[8]

One study found that fructose produces significantly higher blood levels of triglycerides in men.[9] This does not mean you should stop eating whole fruit. The amount of fructose present in natural fruit is small compared to the amount you receive from a glass of regular soda.

In 1981, aspartame was approved for use in foods. You know it by the brand names of NutraSweet and Equal. Diet sodas account for over 70% of the consumption of this product. Yet it is also in over 7,000 other products. Aspartame is a synthetic composite of three naturally occurring compounds: aspartic acid (40%), phenylalanine (50%), and methanol (10%).

Aspartame accounts for over 75% of adverse reactions reported to the FDA annually.[10] Although aspartic acid is a naturally-occurring amino acid, it does have negative consequences in excess.

Too much aspartic acid overstimulates your nerve cells to death. This happens by allowing too much calcium into the cells. Nerve-cell death contributes to a number of chronic illnesses including Alzheimer's disease, brain tumors, dementia, epilepsy, and Parkinson's disease.

Methanol is highly toxic. It breaks down into formic acid and formaldehyde in your body. Some of the symptoms associated with methanol poisoning from aspartame use are:

headaches	nausea	depression
dizziness	chills	fatigue
vertigo	vision problems	anxiety
memory loss	joint pain	sleep disturbances
hearing loss	seizures	heart palpitations

In 1988 the FDA approved acesulfame-potassium (Ace-K) for use. I did not find any reports of adverse reactions. But this product is often blended with aspartame which, as you just learned, has plenty.

Sugar alcohols are another popular alternative. There are five: maltitol, mannitol, sorbitol, isolmalt, and xylitol. All of them are derived from dextrose. Sugar alcohols are the sweeteners in many chewing gums, candies, and dietetic foods. Sugar alcohols can cause intestinal discomfort and diarrhea in some people.

And if you are diabetic, using these products may not be very helpful. There is a nominal difference of carbohydrate grams and calories between sugar and no-sugar varieties of cookies. For the most part, it is the total amount of carbohydrates eaten that will influence glucose (blood sugar) levels in someone with diabetes, not just the amount of simple sugar.[11]

In 1998 sucralose was approved by the FDA. You know sucralose by the brand name Splenda. Sucralose is chlorinated sugar. Consuming more chlorine is definitely not desirable. Research in animals has shown that sucralose can cause many problems in rats, mice, and rabbits, such as[12]:

- Shrunken thymus glands (up to 40% shrinkage)
- Enlarged liver and kidneys
- Atrophy of lymph follicles in the spleen and thymus
- Reduced growth rate
- Decreased red blood cell count
- Diarrhea

Splenda also contains small amounts of lead, arsenic, and methanol.

Satisfy Your Sweet Tooth Naturally

If you find you have any of the aforementioned symptoms, take a break from any products that contain sugar substitutes for 60 days. My research indicates symptoms will subside if you abstain.

When it comes to enjoying sweets, moderation is the rule. I see nothing wrong with indulging your sweet tooth now and again. But having said that, I do think it is important to enjoy foods as they appear naturally.

Natural Flavors: You should try to enjoy the natural taste of foods without trying to make everything sweet. Taste before you sweeten. This will help you develop a more natural palate.

Sugar: If you want to sweeten with sugar, choose brown over white sugar. Also choose sugar "in the raw" over refined. Researchers at Duke University believe sugar has been given an unfair bad rap. And I agree.

Alternative Flavors: Your taste buds do crave other flavors than sweet. Try seasoning your food with sea salt, pepper, basil, oregano, cumin, and thyme to awaken your taste buds.

Alternative Natural Sweeteners: Fruit and honey are nature's candy. Consider adding blueberries or raisins to sweeten your favorite dish. I love using berries because they are low glycemic. I like to enhance the flavor of my tea with slices of oranges, lemons, and limes. I also enjoy eating papayas as a delicious dessert.

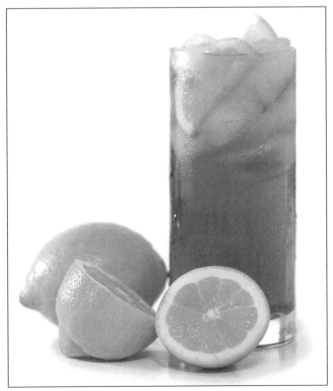

Stevia: As you know, I am very fond of utilizing herbs. There is a naturally sweet plant that I think is a safe alternative. Stevia is a shrubby plant from Paraguay. Its leaves are much sweeter than table sugar and it is calorie free. The FDA has been very resistant to approving stevia as a food additive.

The FDA continues to prefer synthetic creations to naturally occurring plants. You can buy stevia in powdered and liquid form from your health food store. There are great recipes using stevia available at www.stevia.net/recipes.htm.

In the next chapter we'll take a closer look at protein and how it can speed up your metabolism and burn fat.

References:

1 Rabast U., et al. Dietetic treatment of obesity with low and high carbohydrate diets: comparative studies and clinical results. Int J Obes 1979; 3(3): 201-11

2 Lijnen R., et al. Nutritionally induced obesity is attenuated in transgenic mice overexpressing plasminogen activator inhibitor-1. Arter Thromb Vasc Bio 2003; 23: 78-84

3 Herring J. Sold to the Highest Bidder – The Fatally Flawed Food Pyramid. Early to Rise, Mess. #1423. May 25, 2005.

4 Hwang, G, MD, Lee, D, MD, "Trans-fat: The latest and worst fat on the block," Continuing Medical Education, Vol 27, No 2, Feb, 2005:49-54

5 Severson, K, Warner, M, "Fat Substitue is Pushed Out of the Kitchen", The New York Times. Feb 13, 2005: 23.

6 Van Horn Beth "Cooking with Sugar Substitutes" Centre Daily Times, May 3, 2002.

7 Squires, Sally. "Sweet but Not So Innocent?" Washington Post, March 11, 2003: HE01.

8 Squires, Sally. "Sweet but Not So Innocent?" Washington Post, March 11, 2003: HE01.

9 Ibid.

10 Mercola, Joseph "Aspartame: What You Don't Know Can Hurt You"
    http://www.mercola.com/article/aspartame/dangers.htm

11 "Sugar Free Shortcomings for People with Diabetes, Sugar-free Cookies are Not a Free Ride", Tuft's University Health & Nutrition Letter, June 2003.
    http://healthletter.tufts.edu/issues/2003-06/sugar_free.html

12 Mercola, Joseph. "The Potential Dangers of Sucralose"
    http://www.mercola.com/2000/dec/3/sucralose_dangers.htm

Chapter 4
Of What Are You Made?

Your bathroom scale can be misleading. Your total weight doesn't give you a real sense of your progress – or lack of it…

And your government doesn't make it any easier. They use an outdated system called the BMI or Body Mass Index.

In this chapter, I'll show you why BMI doesn't work, what you should use instead, and how you can accurately measure it yourself. It's simple to learn and takes just a few minutes.

Who You Calling Fat?

The BMI is a calculation based on height and weight. But it has one big flaw… <u>It doesn't differentiate fat from muscle</u>.

Because it is so nonspecific, it means almost nothing. Forget about BMI and don't sweat the scale weight either.

Since muscle is denser than fat, it will increase your BMI score more than fat will. And this failure exposes the BMI measurement to a huge potential for error. My own BMI calculates to 29. This would lead you to believe that I am overweight, almost obese. Yet I have only 15% body fat.

Under the BMI system, people with a lot of muscle will have a higher score and will be considered "overweight" (BMI score of 25 to 29.9) or "obese" (BMI score above 30), even though they may be extremely fit.

According to the BMI, these celebrities are "overweight"[1]:

Celebrity	Height	Weight	BMI Score
Michael Jordon	6' 6"	216	25
Will Smith	6' 2"	210	27
George Clooney	5' 11"	211	29

I bet these Hollywood insiders never realized they were "obese."

Celebrity	Height	Weight	BMI Score
Mel Gibson	5' 9"	214	32
Arnold Schwarzenegger	6' 2"	257	33
Sylvester Stallone	5' 9"	228	34

So what is the solution to finding your meaningful measurement for how fit or fat you are?

Use your **body composition**. This measures how much of your weight is fat and how much is lean body mass. The ratio of fat to lean body mass is your real measurement of health.

Men should have 10 to 20% body fat and women should have 15 to 25%. There is little point in measuring more than once every two weeks. Once a month is usually enough for most people.

As you focus on your fat loss goals, aim to <u>increase lean body mass and reduce body fat</u>.

Let the Calipers Set the Record Straight...

There is a simple tool that measures your body composition… a caliper. I generally use three steps when calculating body composition with my patients.

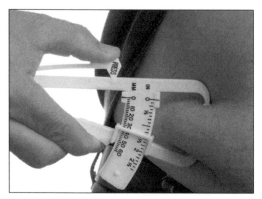

The first step is measuring three different skin folds with your caliper and recording them. A skin fold is what you get when you pinch your skin with your thumb and index finger. (Where you pinch yourself is different for men and women.) Each skin fold is measured in millimeters.

Your second step is adding up the three skin folds to find the sum of your skin folds. This number is also in millimeters.

Your third step is using the slide rule to determine your total body fat based on this total number.

Here's an example:

Body Composition for "John"							
Date	Weight	Chest	Abdomen	Thigh	Sum of Skin Folds	% of Fat	Lbs of Fat	Lean Body Mass
3/01/07	232	37 mm	43 mm	39 mm	119 mm	34.5%	80	152

In this example from one of my patients, I first recorded his weight. I then took three measurements with my calipers. The first was the chest. With John standing up straight and relaxed, I pinched the side of his pectoral muscle (chest). I put my calipers on the pinched skin fold. The reading was 37 mm.

I did the same for his abdomen (in the front, just above the waist). The reading was 43 mm. Then I had John shift his weight onto his left leg and relax his right thigh. I then pinched a skin fold right on top of his thigh. The reading was 39 mm.

Then I added up all three readings: 37 + 43 + 39 = 119 mm. With my slide rule, I positioned the center box, "sum of skin folds" to read "119 to 121."

Since John is a male between the ages of 43 and 47, my slide rule gave me the number 34.5. This is John's percentage of body fat.

Then, I simply took out my calculator and multiplied his weight by 34.5% to determine how many pounds of fat he was carrying. In this case, he had 80 pounds of fat. When you subtract 80 from his weight of 232, you find that he had 152 pounds of lean body mass.

For women, two of the measurements are different.

Instead of measuring the chest, you pinch the area called the "iliac crest." Measuring from the back, this is just above your hip on either side.

Instead of measuring the abdomen, the second measurement for women is the triceps. Simply pinch the back of your arm between your shoulder and your elbow.

For an easier "at home" way to measure your body fat percentage, you take one measurement with your caliper that is approximately one inch above your right hipbone. You take the measurement (in millimeters) and refer to the chart that comes with it. You look for the column where your measurement intersects with your age, and that is your body fat percentage.

Another method of measuring fat is the circumference measurement. This is a useful approximation method using your waist and hip measurements.

Simply wrap a tape measure around your waist at your navel and record the number in inches. Next, measure the circumference around your hips at the widest point. You want your waist to measure at least 1 inch less than your hips.

Now you know the best ways to measure your fat loss progress. See how simple it is? So you are now ready to get started.

In the next chapter we'll look at the first step to changing your eating for fat loss – boosting your metabolism with protein.

References:

1 McKay, Betsy. "Who you calling fat?", Palm Beach Post, July 31, 2002: 1D.

Chapter 5

Step One – Power Up Your Metabolism with Protein

Protein is the only daily essential macronutrient. Fat is also essential, but you can survive longer without fat than you can without protein. Carbohydrates, the third macronutrient, are completely unessential to your diet. In other words, your body can make whatever carbs it needs on its own.

Quality protein is your single most important nutritional concern. It's composed of 20 amino acids, eight of which you can't make and must consume. To be optimally healthy, you must consume all eight of these essential amino acids every day.

Protein is an important component of every cell in your body. Hair and nails are mostly made of protein. Your body uses protein to build and repair tissues. You also use protein to make enzymes, hormones, and other body chemicals. Protein is an important building block of bones, muscles, cartilage, skin, and blood.

But unlike fat and carbohydrates, the body does not store protein, and therefore has no reserve to draw on when it needs a new supply.

Protein Programs Your Body to Burn Fat

As mentioned in chapter 1, overconsuming protein actually programs your body to burn fat. It throws a "metabolic switch" and tells your body that it's okay to burn fat.

Here's why: Your body is not a machine. It's a living, sentient being that makes decisions based on the challenges it faces everyday.

Your body's number one priority is survival. And protein is your body's most prized power source. Under normal circumstances, your body keeps fat on reserve for one reason: to prevent starvation.

But when your body has more protein than it needs, its survival is not threatened. It then feels safe enough to start burning off its fat stores.

Overconsuming protein is one of the easiest, most reliable ways of triggering high-speed fat loss. In addition, you'll guarantee your body has the building blocks it needs for optimum health.

Here's an easy rule-of-thumb for knowing how much protein you need every day: <u>Consume one gram of protein for every pound of lean body mass</u>.

In chapter 4, you measured both your fat and lean body mass. If you weigh 200 pounds and have 20% body fat, that means you're carrying 40 pounds of fat, with 160 pounds of lean body mass. In this example, you would eat 160 grams of protein each day.

This is more than your government recommends. But that's the point… If you're only getting 30 to 60 grams of protein a day, you'll survive – but your body will hold on to its fat for dear life. Overconsume protein and your body responds by dumping fat.

What's more, you'll build powerful muscles that will help you stay mobile and independent far into old age.

To get an extra boost of protein, make protein powder a regular part of your day. The most powerful supplements have **whey protein**. And the best whey protein powders use **whey protein isolate**. This is the most powerful and absorbable form of any protein supplement. Your body can use it right away, and little is wasted.

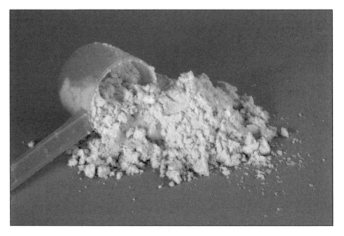

And remember, there were no fat cavemen. They were master hunters who thrived on eating meat – one of the best sources of protein.

Powerful Protein Comes from Animals

We rate proteins by how complete they are. <u>A complete protein contains all of the essential amino acids in the correct ratios</u>. As you can see from the following chart, animal derived foods have the very best protein ratings.[1]

Food	Protein Rating
Eggs	100
Fish	70
Beef	69
Milk	60
Nuts	48
Soybeans	47
Whole wheat	44
Beans	34
Potatoes	34

Eggs are the only source of protein that has a completeness rating of 100 because they have every amino acid in exactly the ratio you require. This is one reason you have heard my recommendations to eat eggs frequently.

Eggs also have only 75 calories, 5 grams of fat, and no trans fats. They also contain 13 essential vitamins and minerals.

A University of Washington study concluded that people with and without high blood cholesterol levels are better off if they eat two eggs a day.[2] Eggs contain the "good fats" that are heart healthy.

Eggs are rich in the nutrient lutein. This nutrient protects against thickening of the arteries. The Los Angeles Atherosclerosis Study found that the more eggs their subjects ate, the better their arteries looked.[3] Eggs have more lutein than a large serving of vegetables.

Aside from being an inexpensive and top-quality source of protein, eggs are filling. You can satiate your appetite and help your brain focus by starting each day with a couple of eggs. I buy organic free-range eggs.

What Are You Really Eating?

But even if you follow a no-grain diet, the meat you buy from the grocery store has been fed grain. The meat industry selects grains because they are very cheap and very fattening. The high glycemic index of corn and other grains induces over-secretion of insulin making the animals enormously fat. This is just like the effect that a grain diet has on us. Then we eat those unnaturally raised and diseased animals. If the cow is diseased, how can we expect to stay healthy by eating it?

Now let me clarify my point. The meat you are eating may be giving you health problems. It has the wrong kind of fat that's unhealthy for your heart. But, contrary to what you hear, this is <u>not because it's red meat</u>. In fact, I regard some beef as among the healthiest of all foods.

There is a difference between grain-fed and grass-fed cattle. To understand the difference, you must understand commercial meat production.

The Problem: Commercial Meat Production

Cattle, in one form or another have been on this planet for millions of years. They have successfully survived by grazing on grasslands, prairies, and hillsides. Cattle's natural diet consists of grasses and legumes. Their anatomy and physiology reflect their diet.

Most commercial cattle no longer eat their natural diet. Growers feed them cheap grain and other "feedstuff" in order to fatten them up quickly. The feedstuffs include hormones to make livestock larger. Ranchers even give the animals antibiotics to keep them alive in deplorable living conditions.

What Your Food Eats[4]	
Commercial Cattle	**Grass-fed Cattle**
Grains, pesticides, hormones, antibiotics, cement dust, candy, animal manure, cardboard, nut shells, feathers, and meat scraps	Pasture Grass Plants

The old saying "you are what you eat" comes to mind. As a result, commercial beef has drastically less nutritional value than that from its pasture-fed relatives. A study in the November 2000 issue of the *Journal of Animal Science* found that the more grass cattle ate, the more nutritious their beef became.[5]

Grass-fed products have three to five times more conjugated linoleic acid (CLA) than that of commercial animals.[6] CLA is an important nutrient that has cancer-preventing properties. Grass-fed beef also has four times more vitamin E.[7]

Omega-3 fatty acids are important to your health. Even more important is the ratio of omega-6 fatty acids to omega-3 fatty acids. Too much omega-6 fatty acids has been linked to heart disease, cancer, and other health problems.

Comparison of Beef Omega 6:3	
Grain-fed beef	20:1
Grass-fed beef	0.16:1

Midwest Land Grant University, August 2001

The Most Complete Nutrition

In our natural environment, approximately 85% of our total calories came from red meat. Red meat is the highest quality nutrition – bar none. In our modern world though, if you eat any animal you have to concern yourself with the environment of that animal. It makes a great deal of difference.

The Solution: Eat Range-Fed

Some grocery stores are starting to offer grass-fed beef. You can ask the butcher. The surest way to get grass-fed products is through a private farm.

New York Times best-selling author Jo Robinson is an aficionado of grass-fed beef. She has compiled a comprehensive list of grass-fed farmers in both the U.S. and Canada. You can access the list by visiting her website www.eatwild.com. Or you can search the Internet for grass-fed farmers such as www.grasslandbeef.com. The beef is delivered to your doorstep packed in ice in a matter of days.

But don't be fooled by beef labeled organic. The organic label only means that the cattle do not have detectable levels of antibiotics or hormones in their body at the time of slaughter. It does not mean that ranchers have never subjected cattle to antibiotics or hormones. Also, most organic cattle eat nutritionally deficient grains.

Grass-fed meat is a deep red to maroon color, not pink like commercial beef. And grass-fed beef is very lean. The flavor is richer and tastes like wild game.

The USDA and Your Food Labels

Products may display very ambiguous labels that deceive most consumers. A few common and misleading labels are "cage free" and "free range". These phrases are not well defined, so manufacturers can use them as they see fit.

The "cage free" is a label on poultry and eggs. But "cage free" only means that the manufacturer did not confine poultry in an individual cage. Dozens of chickens are bound in a pen with no room to move, and the "cage free" label is still be used.

"Free range" means that an animal has access to the outdoors for an unspecified period of time everyday. Individual manufacturers regulate this time period. This means that a door could be open to the outside for a few minutes a day. Whether or not the animal goes outside is irrelevant. The manufacturer can still use the "free range" label.

Look for the USDA "Free Farmed" label on poultry, dairy, and eggs. And the USDA "Grass Fed" label on beef. These labels are well defined and verified by the USDA. If you cannot find these products in the supermarket, buy from a private farmer. They are more nutritious and do not carry hormones and antibiotics.

What You Need to Know About Mad Cow Disease

Mad Cow disease, also known as bovine spongiform encephalopathy (BSE) is, as far as we know, a relatively new disease. The disease eats holes in the brains of infected cows. Humans can contract a variant if they eat infected beef.

Mad cow is spread by cannibalism. Cows can get it if they ingest cow flesh. How can that ever happen? Well, modern ranchers don't publicize it, but they have been intentionally feeding cattle cow parts for years. To cut costs they grind up cow body parts that no one else wants and mix them back into the cattle feed.

Cows are herbivores. Animal parts have no place in their diets. This disease doesn't exist in their natural environment. It is a product of the meat-producing industry. Only if a cow eats cow parts can it develop Mad Cow disease.

There is no treatment but prevention is simple. Stop the macabre practice of feeding cattle cow parts. Don't import cattle from anywhere that does. The case occurring in the first cow in the U.S. is evidence of failure of our only defense – prevention.

When our government repeatedly insisted the U.S. was different, that it just couldn't happen here, I couldn't help but be puzzled. Why not? Each

European country claimed it had preventative measures in place as well. One by one, they fell to Mad Cow like dominos. What was so different here? During this time American cattle had the same cannibalistic feeding practice. The FDA insisted stricter measures were not necessary.

It now appears they didn't happen because of heavy lobbying by the powerful meat producing industry. The FDA and USDA comments were more directed at the international beef trade on behalf of the U.S. food industry than to the U.S. beef consumer. For whatever reason, one thing is sure – the USDA, the FDA, and the CDC failed in this simple prevention despite a decade and a half of repeated assurances to the contrary.

Eat Grass-Fed Beef for Peace of Mind and Better Nutrition

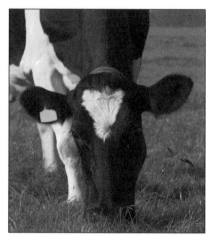

You don't have to give up your prime rib. Simply choose grass-fed beef only. Since these cattle eat only their natural diet of range grass Mad Cow is never a concern. You won't have to rely on the government that failed to stop it in cattle. The added bonus is you will be eating a higher quality protein packed with CoQ10 and with more omega-3 (good) than omega-6 (bad) fats. Beef is also the best source of the B vitamins.

Overcooking Your Meat Puts You at Risk for Chronic Disease

Do you love steak that's nice and pink in the middle? Me too… But conventional wisdom says it's "dangerous." So let me put your mind at ease.

The idea that it's "healthier" to cook meat until it's dry and tasteless is no more than an urban legend. It's not based on scientific fact. And cooking your food that way can cause arthritis, cancer, diabetes, and heart disease.

Overcooking food is a bad idea. It denatures protein, breaks down vitamins, and removes nutrients. Many cooking techniques that achieve a high temperature trigger a chemical change that mimics aging. New studies have linked eating these foods to premature aging and a host of chronic diseases.

Imagine overcooked food. It becomes dry, wrinkled, hard, blistered, and discolored. That same process is occurring in your body each time you consume foods cooked improperly.

What I'm talking about here is the process of *glycation*. Glycation is what happens to the proteins in our body as we age. The same process turns a turkey's skin brown and crispy when it's cooked.

Glycation is really the binding of protein and glucose molecules. The result is a spoiled protein assembly. These deviants are *glycotoxins*. And glycotoxins are responsible for accelerated aging and disease.

As the glycotoxins accumulate in your cells, they send out chemical signals. The body responds by producing sites of inflammation. In addition, the abnormal protein structures do not regenerate. They remain damaged. This is the process of aging and disease.

When we cook foods at high temperatures, large amounts of glycotoxins collect in the food. A new study demonstrated that if we eat these foods, the glycotoxins transfer to our tissues.

Researchers at the Mt. Sinai School of Medicine evaluated 24 diabetic participants. Scientists split the subjects into two groups. One group ate a diet low in glycotoxins. The other group ate a diet high in glycotoxins.

After only two weeks, the group eating the high-glycotoxin diet had up to 100% more glycotoxins present in their blood and urine than those who ate the low-glycotoxin diet.[8]

This is clear evidence that the glycotoxins from your food transfer into your body.

Overcooking has another negative consequence. It denatures many important nutrients in food. One of the best examples is CoQ10. You need

CoQ10 for proper functioning of all of the major organs in your body. The best source of CoQ10 is red meat. Overcooking meat destroys CoQ10. Just by changing a few cooking habits, you can enjoy good food, without the danger. And you can add a supplement to your routine that helps fight glycation.

High-heat cooking methods usually cause food to change color or consistency. We like this kind of cooking because it makes the food tasty. But if you want to avoid premature aging, try some different techniques:

Fight Glycation by Changing Your Habits...	
Avoid:	Try this Instead:
Fried	Steam
Microwaved	Stew
Broiled	Boiling
Charred	Poaching

You can reduce the number of glycotoxins in your food by cooking it at a lower heat. But low heat doesn't have to be low in taste. You can use spices and fresh herbs to boost the taste of meals cooked at lower heat. Marinating your meat before you cook it is another good way to prevent or slow glycation.

The only supplement proven to prevent glycation is *carnosine*. A recent laboratory study shows that carnosine actually plays a role in disposing of glycated proteins in your tissues.[9] About 1000-mg of carnosine daily should protect your body from being cooked from the inside, out. Carnosine also protects your muscles from degenerating.

Eat Like Our Ancestors and Prevent Chronic Disease

Eat a diet similar to our stone-age ancestors and you'll avoid most modern diseases.

Cavemen ate what they could hunt or gather. Their archeological record combined with studies of modern hunters shows virtually no heart disease, diabetes, osteoarthritis, or obesity. To enjoy this native good health in our day and age, start by eating what they ate – whole foods consisting of natural meats and eggs, true vegetables, unmodified fruits and real nuts, and olives.

Man ate only whole foods for a millennia. Factory-produced foods have only recently become a staple. Food additives such as aspartame, high fructose corn syrup, and hydrogenated vegetable oils are in almost all packaged supposed health foods. Heart disease, diabetes, and obesity have coincided with these dietary changes. Prior to the agricultural revolution, these chronic diseases were rare.

There are remote populations today that still adhere to a hunter-gatherer diet. In these populations, the elderly people are generally free of the chronic diseases (obesity, high blood pressure, heart disease) that almost universally afflict the elderly in modern societies.[10]

When these people adopt western diets, their health declines, and they begin to exhibit the same signs and symptoms of the diseases in our civilization today. Your body is an amazing, adaptable machine, but straying too far from your natural diet makes your health suffer.

Many people question the wisdom of caveman eating because cavemen didn't live as long as most people do today. But understand that trauma, predation, and infection caused most early deaths in hunter-gatherer societies. If an individual was fortunate to avoid these dangers, for as long as he lived, he was free of the chronic degenerative diseases that afflict modern societies.

Surprising to most of my patients, cavemen ate more protein and fat than modern Americans do. But … they ate a whole lot less carbohydrate. They ate no processed carbohydrates and no fat derived from vegetable oils.

Protein and natural fats with fruits and vegetables that you can eat as you grow lays a strong foundation for health. That's what cavemen ate and it's what you should eat.

Following are some of these ancient foods.

Nature's Sweetest Cancer Fighters

Blueberries are an amazing food with a long list of benefits. Starting at the top of your body, eating blueberries is a gift to your brain. The natural dye anthocyanin that gives blueberries their color protects brain cells. Also, the antioxidants in blueberries calm inflammation. Together, these chemicals are responsible 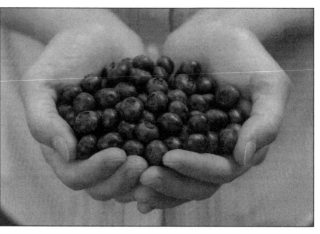 for protecting against short-term memory loss. A team at Tufts University pinpointed these chemicals after showing that mice and people performed better on motor skill tests after eating a serving of blueberries a day.[11]

Eating blueberries also helps prevent cancer. A group at the University of Illinois explained that anthocyanins inhibit the initiation and promotion of cancer in your body. The antioxidants in blueberries, such as ellagic acid, make you three times less likely to develop cancer than people that don't eat them.[12]

The list of good blueberry qualities goes on.

Looking to avoid heart disease? Eat blueberries! Just a half-pint of blueberries contains five grams of dietary fiber. A Harvard study concluded that men with a high fiber intake were at a 40% lower risk of heart disease.[13]

An eye specialist in La Jolla, California, found that patients who ate blueberries had a marked improvement in their eyesight. This has led researchers to look at blueberries as a medicine to ward off macular degeneration.[14]

Convenient Snacks Packaged by Nature

And here's some more good news to crunch on: Nuts are another super healthy food that will help raise the good cholesterol in your body and provide you with plenty of fiber as well as reduce your risk of disease.

A Harvard School of Public Health study reported that eating five or more 1-ounce servings of nuts each week reduced the participants' risk of Type 2 diabetes by nearly 30%.

Even the much-maligned peanut butter got a good review – eating five tablespoons of peanut butter each week reduced the diabetes risk by almost 20%.[15]

Nuts had a bad reputation for a long time because they are full of fat. But, like eggs, the fat in nuts is healthy, monounsaturated fat. In addition, nuts provide a wide variety of heart-disease-fighting vitamins and minerals such as vitamin E (a potent antioxidant), folic acid, niacin, magnesium, vitamin B_6, zinc, copper, and potassium. And the list goes on – nuts also contain the nonessential amino acid arginine, which can protect the inner lining of the arterial walls.[16]

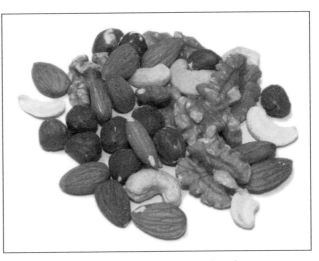

So go ahead and stock up the nut dish with peanuts, pecans, walnuts, and almonds!

An Ancient Food that Lowers Your Cholesterol Naturally

If you're looking to lower your cholesterol and reduce your risk of heart disease and cancer, then pop an olive in your mouth. A Harvard study showed that eating monounsaturated fats like olives lowers your risk for heart disease. These good fats lower LDL and raise HDL cholesterol levels. They also prevent the build-up of plaque on your artery walls.[17]

The olive contains monounsaturated fats and antioxidants. They are also high in vitamins A, K, and E. And they have a high proportion of the essential amino acids. Yes, another near perfect, true health food – and just the right size for snacking!

Let Spicy Food Be Your Medicine

Cayenne is a perfect example of the old maxim, "The sheer magnitude of health benefits in cayenne peppers is astounding." Their fiery heat fends off ailments such as heart disease, cancers, cataracts, and Alzheimer's disease. Hot red peppers also help heal the common cold and flu. They can even stop internal and external bleeding.

The main medical properties of cayenne come from a chemical called capsaicin, that gives peppers their heat. Generally, the hotter the pepper, the more capsaicin contains and the healthier it is for your body.

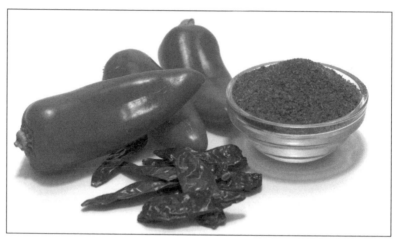

Cultures that regularly use hot peppers like cayenne have a much lower rate of heart attack, stroke, and pulmonary embolism. This is because cayenne peppers improve circulation. They cut the mucus in the venous system, which facilitates blood flow throughout the body.

Capsaicin is a potent inhibitor of substance P, a neuropeptide associated with inflammatory processes. The research shows that peppers can help control sensory nerve fiber disorders, including pain associated with arthritis, psoriasis, and diabetic neuropathy.[18]

So, start heating up those Cajun recipes, and get your heart healthy.

In the next chapter Step Two will further help you fight fat by providing you with a guide to expose the unwanted carbs hiding in your diet.

References:

1 Agatston, Arthur. Drop13 Pounds in 14 Days: "A Crash Course in the South Beach Diet Program, by the cardiologist who made losing weight taste great" Men's Health, September 2003: 112-114.

2 Knopp, et. Al., University of Washington Study, Journal of American College of Clinical Nutrition 1997; 65:1747-64.

3 Dwyer et al., The Los Angeles Atherosclerosis Study, Circulation 2001; 103:2922-2977.

4 Robinson J. Why Grassfed is Best Vashon Island Press: WA 2000, pg. 10

5 French P, et al. Fatty acid composition, including conjugated linoleic acid, of intramuscular fat from steers offered grazed grass, grass silage, or concentrate-based diets. J Anim Sci 2000; 78: 2849-2855

6 Dhiman T, et al. Conjugated linoleic acid from cows fed different diets. J Dairy Sci 1999; 82(10): 2146-2156

7 Smith G. Dietary supplementation of Vitamin E to cattle to improve shelf life and case life of beef for domestic and international markets. Colorado State University.

8 Vlassara H., et al. Inflammatory mediators are induced by dietary glycotoxins, a major risk factor for diabetic angiopathy. Proc Natl Acad Sci USA 2003 Jan 21; 100(2): 763.

9 Yeargans G., et al. Carnosine promotes the heat denaturation of glycated protein. Biochem Biophys Res Commun 2003 Jan 3; 300(1): 75-80

10 Cordain L et al. "Plant animal subsistence ratios and macronutrient energy estimates in worldwide hunter-gatherer diets." The American Journal of Clinical Nutrition, 2000 Mar; 71(3): 682-692

11 Journal of Neuroscience, 1999 Sep; 19 (18):8114-8121.

12 Journal of Food Science, 2000; 65(2).

13 Harvard School of Public Health – Fiber, http://www.hsph.harvard.edu/nutritionsource/fiber.html

14 Superfoods' Everyone Needs, by G. Shaw, Feb 2, 2004

15 Journal of the American Medical Association, Nov 27, 2002.

16 http://www.clevelandclinic.org/heartcenter/pub/guide/prevention/nutrition/nuts.htm

17 John Stark. "Olives", Body and Soul, April 2004

18 Todd C./ Meeting the therapeutic challenge of the patient with osteoarthiritis. J Am Pharm Assoc (Wash) 2002; 42:74-82.

Chapter 6

Step Two – Try This Simple Carb Tester

Change your carbohydrate and you can trump up fat burning. It doesn't have to be difficult or involve a great deal of sacrifice. But most "experts" miss the real point and recommend unnecessary and less effective restriction.

Here's the big point: When you're considering which carbs to avoid, it's not about sugar or sweetness… It's about "starchiness." Starches have the highest scores on the glycemic index. And that's what really matters when it comes to burning off your fat.

The *glycemic index* (GI) measures how the carbohydrates in foods increase your blood sugar. Foods with a high GI will spike your blood sugar. Foods with a low GI have carbohydrates that break down slowly, releasing a more manageable trickle of glucose into your bloodstream.[1]

Why is this so critical to body fat?

When your blood sugar rises, it triggers a release of the hormone insulin. Too much insulin is not a problem just for diabetics. It's a concern for you, too. Insulin's role in normal metabolism is to handle blood sugar **and build body fat**.

All other things being equal, more insulin tells your body to store more of the calories you consume as body fat.

Here's the result in its simplest form: **Excess insulin makes you fat.**

Blood sugar is the most basic form of "food" for your cells. And one of the jobs of insulin is to bring blood sugar into your cells. In this regard, insulin is a kind of transportation service. Without insulin, the nourishment your cells need would never arrive.

But I think of hormones as "double-edged swords." Either too much and too little can cause big problems. And when you repeatedly eat high-glycemic foods, your body repeatedly sends more insulin into your bloodstream.

Over time your body becomes less and less responsive to insulin. As this happens, your body has to secrete more and more insulin to get the job done. This leads to a condition called ***insulin resistance***. This continues and you're fat, tired, and headed for chronic disease.

There are also many other related problems: As a reaction to the rapid release of insulin, your blood sugar will often crash – just as quickly as it spiked from the high GI food. This sudden drop of blood sugar will make you crave the same foods that spiked your blood sugar in the first place.

If you're not watching your diet, this cycle repeats endlessly. Before you know it, you're packing on pound after pound of unwanted fat.

What foods are the worst offenders? Breakfast cereals, bagels, breads, white rice, and potatoes have some of the highest GI scores. Not sweets but starches.

Meat, fish, poultry, eggs and nuts continue to be some of the best foods you can eat. They are very low on the glycemic index – so enjoy that steak.

Plain yogurt and most kinds of fruit are also excellent choices. The sweetness you taste from berries is a guilt-free pleasure because the total load of carbs will be low and they rank very low on the glycemic index.

I've included a comprehensive glycemic index on the next page… I put this list together with research from my Wellness Research Foundation. It will give you all the latest numbers and avoid the bias over sweets so common in other lists.

First, a few pointers: The index is expressed in percentage terms. For example, foods with a glycemic index of 50 will cause your blood sugar to rise ***half*** as much as glucose (pure blood sugar).

Foods with a glycemic index of 100 will cause your blood sugar to rise ***the same*** as pure glucose. Foods with a glycemic index of zero will not raise your blood sugar at all.

You may be surprised to hear this, but rarely a food can have a GI score higher than 100. That means it spikes your blood sugar **more** than pure glucose. Corn bread is the best example.

Remember… The higher the glycemic index, the more fat you'll make from that food. Even if it has an equal number of calories.

For high-speed fat loss, keep most of your choices below 40.

FOOD	SCORE	FOOD	SCORE
GLYCEMIC INDEX			
GRAIN PRODUCTS			
Corn Bread	110	Couscous	65
Instant rice	91	Quick Oats Instant Porridge	65
Corn chips	72	Basmati white rice	58
Millet	71	Whole-wheat pita	57
Corn tortilla	70	White rice	56
Corn meal	68	Corn (sweet)	55
Rye crackers	68	Oatmeal, old fashioned	48
Taco shell	68	Bulgur	48
Stoned wheat thins	67	Barley	25
CEREAL			
Kellogg's Corn Flakes	92	Instant Cream of Wheat	74
Rice Chex	89	Shredded Wheat	67
Kellogg's Crispix	87	Cream of Wheat	66
Corn Chex	83	Quick Oats Life	66
Rice Krispies	82	Life	66
Kellog's Rice Krispies	82	Kellog's Raisin Bran	61
Corn Pops	80	Mini Shredded Wheats	58
Grapenuts flakes	80	Bran Chex	58
Grapenuts	75	Muesli	56
Total	76	Frosted Flakes	55
Cheerios	74	Kellogg's Special K	54
Puffed wheat	74	All Bran	51

FOOD	SCORE	FOOD	SCORE
BREAD			
French baguette	95	Hamburger buns	61
Pretzels	81	Cheese pizza	60
Kaiser roll	73	Bran muffin	60
Bagel	72	Blueberry muffin	59
White bread	70	Pita	57
Melba Toast	70	Sourdough	54
Whole-wheat bread	69	Oat and raisin bread	54
American rye bread	68	Oat bran bread	48
Croissant	67	Banana bread	47
100% whole-rye bread	65	Pumpernickel bread	41
CAKES/COOKIES/CANDIES			
Rice cakes	82	Sara Lee pound cake	54
Jelly beans	80	Pound cake	54
Vanilla Wafers	77	Strawberry jam	51
Graham crackers	74	Chocolate bar	49
Saltine crackers	74	Apple cinnamon	44
Honey	73	Betty Crocker vanilla cake with vanilla frosting	42
Life Savers	70	Snickers bar	41
Flan cake	65	Betty Crocker chocolate cake with frosting	38
Table sugar	65	Fructose	22
Shortbread cookies	64		
PASTA			
Linguine	55	Vermicelli	35
Cheese Tortellini	50	Spaghetti (5 min. boiled)	33
Macaroni	45	Fettuccini	32
Spaghetti (15 min. boiled)	44	Spaghetti (protein enriched)	28
Spaghetti whole wheat	37		

FOOD	SCORE	FOOD	SCORE
BEVERAGES			
Gatorade	78	Nestle hot chocolate mix	51
Ocean Spray cranberry juice cocktail	68	Grapefruit juice	48
Coca Cola	63	Pineapple juice	46
Orange juice-frozen concentrate	57	Apple juice	41
Orange juice-fresh	52	Tomato juice	38
DAIRY / DAIRY SUBSTITUTE			
Tofu frozen dessert	115	Chocolate milk	35
Ice cream	47	Yogurt (low fat, sugar)	33
Pudding	44	Milk (fat free)	32
Custard	43	Whole milk	30
Yogurt (fruit)	36	Yogurt	14
FRUIT			
Watermelon	72	Orange	43
Pineapple	66	Grapes	43
Cantaloupe	65	Strawberries (fresh)	40
Raisins	64	Yogurt (fruit)	36
Apricot (canned in light syrup)	64	Apple	36
Papaya	60	Pear	36
Peaches (canned in heavy syrup)	58	Apricot (dried)	31
Fruit cocktail (drained, Del Monte)	55	Peaches (canned in light syrup)	30
Banana	53	Prunes	29
Kiwi	52	Peach (fresh)	28
Mango	51	Plum	24
Dates	50	Grapefruit	25
Pear (canned in pear juice)	44	Cherries	22

FOOD	SCORE	FOOD	SCORE
NUTRITIONAL-SUPPORT PRODUCTS			
Enercal Plus	61	Choice DM	23
Ensure	50		
MEAL REPLACEMENT BARS			
Kudos whole-grain bars (chocolate)	61	L.E.A.N Nutribar (chocolate crunch)	30
Pure-protein bar (strawberry)	43	L.E.A.N Nutribar (peanut crunch)	30
Pure-protein bar (with chocolate)	40	Pure Protein bar (peanut butter)	22
Pure-protein bar (chocolate deluxe)	38		
POTATOES			
Potato (white, boiled)	104	Mashed potato	73
Red potato (baked)	93	Potato chips	54
Instant mashed potatoes	83	Sweet potato	54
French fries	76	Yam	51
LEGUMES			
Canned green pea soup	66	Lima beans (boiled)	32
Split pea soup with ham	66	Chick peas, boiled	31
Canned black bean soup	64	Marrow gat peas, boiled	31
Canned kidney beans	52	Navy beans, boiled	31
Baked beans	48	Cannellini beans	31
Peas	48	Lentils (green, brown)	30
Green pea (frozen)	47	Lentils	28
Pinto-eyed peas, boiled	45	Red lentils (boiled)	27
Canned chickpeas	45	Kidney beans	23
Lentil soup	44	Dried peas	22
Black eyed peas	42	Soy beans, boiled	20
Butter beans	36	Peanuts	13
Garbanzo beans	34	Beans (string or green)	0
Lima beans (frozen)	32		

FOOD	SCORE	FOOD	SCORE
NUTS			
Cashews	22	Macadamia	0
Almonds	0	Pecans	0
Brazil nuts	0	Walnuts	0
Hazelnuts	0		
VEGETABLES			
Parsnip	97	Eggplant	0
Carrots	92	Snow peas	0
Beets (canned)	64	Artichokes	0
Tomato soup	38	Peppers	0
Tomato	15	Spinach	0
Mushroom	0	Summer squash	0
Broccoli	0	Asparagus	0
Cabbage	0	Cucumber	0
Cauliflower	0	Zucchini	0
Celery	0	Lettuce	0
MEAT / PROTEIN			
Beef	0	Lamb	0
Chicken	0	Pork	0
Eggs	0	Veal	0
Fish	0		

Let's look at a few examples to see how this plays out during everyday life… Let's say you get up in the morning and pour yourself a bowl of Kellogg's Corn Flakes. You've seen the TV commercials telling you that this "nutritious" cereal is packed with vitamins and minerals. So you figure it's healthy, right? Not exactly…

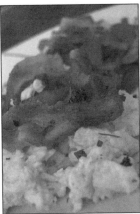

If you look at your GI, Kellogg's Corn Flakes score a 92! That means your blood sugar will fly off the charts almost as quickly as if you'd eaten pure sugar. Not the way you want to start your day.

What if you decided to jump-start your morning with eggs and bacon? Eggs and bacon both score a zero! Your grandparent's generation had it right. Not only will eggs and bacon keep you slim; they give you a nice shot of protein, which is exactly what you need in the morning.

There are other surprises, too… Which will help you burn fat faster, a Snickers Bar or a plain rice cake? Answer: Snickers Bar. It goes against everything you've been taught about diet and nutrition, but rice cakes will make you fat. The starchy rice cake scores an 82 on the GI. A Snicker's Bar is a moderate 41.

You see, the fat in the Snickers Bar works to your advantage. It slows the rise of blood sugar and will actually result in a smaller release of insulin. Ice cream is the same. The fat content gives it a lower GI.

Now don't go overboard… I'm not suggesting you load up on Snicker's Bars and ice cream. Eat enough, and the sugar and extra calories will easily catch up with you. But similarly, don't fool yourself into thinking that a rice cake will help you. It won't.

Whole-wheat bread is another diet trap. Most people think whole wheat is better for you than regular white bread. But look at their GI scores… White bread scores a 70 and whole wheat scores a 69! Almost identical. In terms of fat gain, both kinds of bread are equally unhealthy.

Revitalize Your Fat-Loss Hormone

When you eat sugary and starchy foods, the balance of another important hormone gets thrown out of balance. Leptin, a hormone made from fat cells, is a key player in weight regulation.

Leptin tells your brain how much energy you have and how to use it. When you have enough, leptin tells your brain to stop eating and start burning fat. When your energy is low, leptin tells your brain to increase your appetite so you'll start eating.

New research shows that you can become "leptin resistant" in the same way you can become insulin resistant.[2] When your cells can no longer hear or understand the messages coming from hormones, we say they are resistant.

This happens when too much of the hormone is in the bloodstream for an extended period. In fact, leptin resistance can lead to insulin resistance. This in turn puts you at risk for obesity, heart disease, diabetes, and cancer.

When you eat foods that spike your blood sugar, both insulin and leptin get thrown out of balance. As you know, high blood sugar triggers a surge of insulin. And when that sugar is metabolized in your fat cells, those fat cells release a surge of leptin.

Like "crying wolf," if this surge happens too often, the cells become resistant to leptin's message. As a result, your brain never gets the message that you have enough energy stores to burn fat or control your appetite. It can leave you feeling hungry all the time with the constant temptation to overeat.

In addition to weight regulation, leptin plays a pivotal role in controlling your brain's hypothalamus. This in turn regulates your "autonomic" functions – the ones that happen without you having to think about them.

Expose the Empty Carbs Hiding in Your Diet

Empty carbs are everywhere. Rate your true carb consumption with this little quiz:[3]

1. Do you drink soft drinks, sweetened fruit drinks or punches every day? (If yes, give yourself 3 points.)

2. Do you eat dessert two or more times a week? (If yes, give yourself 3 points.)

3. Do you choose snacks from the vending machine at work two or more times a week? (If yes, give yourself 3 points.)

4. Do you eat canned or frozen fruit? (If yes, give yourself 3 points.)

5. Do you drink "health" teas or energy drinks? (If yes, give yourself 3 points.)

6. Do you eat canned vegetables? (If yes, give yourself 3 points.)

7. Do you eat "meal replacement" or energy bars? (If yes, give yourself 3 points.)

8. Do you add sugar to coffee or tea often? (If yes, give yourself 3 points.)

9. Do you use jam, jelly, or honey on bread or rolls regularly? (If yes, give yourself 3 points.)

Total up your score. If you scored higher than 9, you're at risk for an empty-carb overload.

What can you do? First thing, cut out processed foods entirely. This alone will cut out a lot of your high-glycemic carbs. You'll improve your health and even sleep better at night. All the refined sugar can leave you jittery. Then, replace them with healthier alternatives. I'll show you how in chapter 7.

These include:

- Body temperature
- Heart rate
- Hunger
- Stress response
- Fat burning and storage
- Reproductive behavior
- Bone growth and blood sugar levels

When you realize there's so much more to this pathology than just weight gain, it's no wonder weight gain is associated with so many chronic diseases.

Fortunately, there are simple ways of restoring balance. A new study from a university in Canada shows that exercise and supplementing with fish oil can help your body become sensitive to leptin.[4]

The fish oil puts back essential omega-3 fatty acids into your system. There's more on fish oil in chapter 7.

References:

1 Whyte JJ. The Glycemic Index: How Useful Is It? Peer-Reviewed Consultations in Primary Care. Apr 15, 2005. Vol.45. 558-560.

2 Dyck D. Leptin Sensitivity in Skeletal Muscle Is Modulated by Diet and Exercise. Exerc. Sport Sci. Rev., Vol. 33, No. 4, pp. 189-194, 2005.

3 West/Wadsworth Publishing Company, "Carbohydrate Consumption Scorecard", 2001.

4 Dyck D., pp. 189-194.

Chapter 7

Step Three – Eat the Right Fats to Burn Fat

The right fats can put you in high-speed fat loss mode – especially when you combine them with progressive intensity exercise. In chapter 9, I'll tell you more about how that works and give you a customized fat-burning PACE® routine you can do right away.

Researcher Dr. Peter Howe from the University of South Australia studied overweight to obese people for 12 weeks. He divided them up into groups for a trial that looked at the effect of omega-3 fish oil taken daily in combination with exercise three times a week.

They were compared with three other groups taking just fish oil, just sunflower oil, or a combination of sunflower oil and exercise.

"Our research showed that the fish oil and exercise group lost significantly more fat mass than any other group in the study," reported Dr. Howe.

"Seeing the impact on body shape and body composition of these participants has been the most exciting outcome of the research."

He added: *"Omega-3 fatty acids in fish oil are polyunsaturated fats that can* **switch on enzymes specifically involved in oxidizing or burning of fat,** *but they need a driver (in our case, exercise) to increase the metabolic rate in order to lower body fat."*

This study proves the effectiveness of omega-3s to burn fat. Yet the media still claims that low-fat diets will give you a dream body and protect you from disease.

Finally, New Proof for Old-Fashioned Fats in Your Diet

In 2006, the large-scale Women's Health Initiative study confounded its researchers when it showed that low-fat diets offer no benefit against chronic diseases.[1] In fact, low-fat diets only *increased* risks, especially for diabetes.

This message is hard to get through when billions are spent every year to prove otherwise. Food producers profit more when you fear fat because low-fat carbohydrates from wheat, corn, and soy are much higher profit. And as soon as these findings were released, the spin doctors tried to confuse the public over this very simple and stark finding.

The Women's Health Initiative spent eight years and $415 million studying the diets of 50,000 women. *"Based on our findings, we cannot recommend that most women should follow a low-fat diet."* Those were the words of Jacques Rossouw of the National Heart, Lung and Blood Institute, which financed the study.

This applies to men as well. In fact, no one should eat a low-fat diet. It defies logic, instinctive tastes, good sense, history, nature, fundamental physiological science, and now the best direct prospective, controlled, population study to date.

One of the finest epidemiologists I've ever had the pleasure to meet, Dr. Walter Willett of Harvard University recently put it well. *"It was a mistake, and this study really confirms that it was the wrong direction to go for nutritional advice. This should be the nail in the coffin for low-fat diets."*[2]

Here's more proof: A study published in the *Journal of The American Medical Association* found people eating very low-fat diets showed no improvement in body composition, blood sugar, insulin levels, or blood pressure. In fact, the study's authors called very low-fat diets "counterproductive" to health.[3]

Another problem with low-fat diets is that they are high-carb. Excessive intake of the wrong kinds of carbohydrates, not fat, is the central dietary problem in my patient population. What's more, if you follow all this low-fat advice you could be robbing your body of essential nutrients.

Your body needs fat to absorb vitamins. In fact, some of the most important nutrients, such as vitamins A, D, E, and K and CoQ10, are fat-soluble.

Cut out all the fat and you cut out these essential nutrients.

Is this a license to load up on fatty sausage and processed luncheon meat? Absolutely not. You should be focusing on eating *good* fats and eliminating bad ones if you want to stay young, strong, and the focus of this book – burning off body fat.

Knowing the Good from the Bad… Choose Your Fats Wisely

Here's an easy way of thinking about fats: Divide dietary fat into three groups: Omega-3s, omega-6s, and trans fats. These are the good, the bad, and the ugly of fats.

You should avoid the ugly trans fats and take a little effort to rebalance your good and bad fats. You need omega-3 and omega-6 fatty acids for good health. Your body cannot make enough, so you need to get them from your diet. They're essential for building and maintaining brain tissue.

These fats are also vital structural components of cell membranes. And you use them to make a variety of hormones known as prostaglandins. Both their amount and ratio in the diet have important physiological impacts on your health.

The Good Fat: Omega-3s

Good sources of omega-3s are salmon, avocado, walnuts, olives, and olive oil. Omega-3s, and particularly EPA and DHA, reduce your risk of dying from cardiovascular disease (CVD) and other diseases.

The Bad Fat: Omega-6s

Omega-6s are in animal and plant foods. Although omega-6s are essential to a balanced diet, you only need a modest amount. Too much can cause heart disease, diabetes, obesity, fatigue, inability to concentrate, and memory loss.

The Ugly Fat: Trans Fats

Trans fats lurk in low-fat cookies, cakes, cereal, chips, crackers, and fried fast food like French fries and chicken nuggets. They are a creation of the modern food industry for their convenience. They are the ugly fat that has no place in your diet.

Strike the Right Balance Between Omega-3s and Omega-6s

You're probably not getting enough of the right fats in your diet. But you're not alone. We all have the same problem. Omega-3 and omega-6 fatty acids are essential to life. Your heart and brain depend on them. But the natural levels of omega-3s in your food keep getting lower and lower.

That means you often end up with high levels of omega-6s and a lack of omega-3s. And that causes inflammation, which is at the root of so many health concerns today. Arthritis and heart disease are just to name a few.

Before the days of modern industry, your meat and fish had abundant supplies of omega-3s. But these days, even some salmon has little to none of this essential oil. And that's bad news, because your body can't make omega-3s on its own. And without it, your risk of disease skyrockets.

When your levels are low, you can expect a higher risk of:

- Heart disease
- Stroke
- Diabetes
- Arthritis
- Depression
- Skin disorders
- Macular degeneration

As is often true in nature, balance is essential. Your body needs both omega-3s and omega-6s, <u>but in the right ratios</u>. For most of the time humans have been on Earth, we ate foods that had omega-6s and omega-3s in roughly equal proportion up to a ratio of about 2:1.

Over the last 75 years, omega-6s in our diet have soared. Now the ratio is somewhere about 10:1 with some of my patients eating even 20 times more omega-6s as omega-3s. And the average American eats 10 times the absolute quantity of omega-6s that is healthy. The main sources of omega-6s are vegetable oils, processed foods and grain-fed beef.

That is where the health "gurus" of the 1980s made another big mistake. They mistook the heart disease culprit to be red meat because ***grain-fed***, commercial cattle have the very high 20:1 ratio of omega-6s to omega-3s.

But they never bothered to explain why native cultures, who ate meat from ***grass-fed*** cattle, never had a single case of heart disease.

If you measure omega-6s and omega-3s in wild or grass-fed animals, you get a very different picture. Their ratio is a dramatically reversed – and heart healthy – 0.16 to 1. In other words, the culprit is not the fat in meat. It's the environment in which cattle are raised that changes the ratio of fats in their body.

Grain-fed cattle are sick cattle. They're not supposed to eat grains. It's not natural for them and it changes their physiology. When cattle lose omega-3s, so do we. By eating their meat, we take on the same problems.

Farm-raised fish are the same. Salmon bred under these conditions don't get the chance to live in their natural environment or eat their natural diet. Instead, they're fed "fish flakes." The same kind of stuff you would feed your goldfish at home. And the results are the same: a drastic loss of omega-3 fatty acids.

Aside from eating grass-fed beef and wild salmon – which can get expensive – your best bet to restore natural levels of omega-3 fatty acids is to take a supplement. Certain brands of cod liver oil work best. And they're relatively inexpensive.

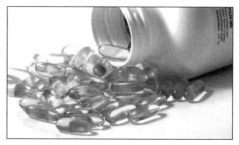

The benefits are practically endless and your body needs a steady supply. Many of my own patients have not only reversed disease but improved their mental and emotional lives as well.

Supplementing with cod liver oil:

• Prevents heart disease, cancer – even strokes

• Lowers your blood pressure

• Wipes out arthritis pain

• Relieves depression

• Lowers triglycerides (blood fat)

• Raises HDL (good cholesterol)

• Boosts your memory and brain power

• Lowers risk of macular degeneration

• Protects your blood vessels and nerves

• Calms irregular heart rhythms, which can lead to sudden cardiac death

Scores of clinical reports back this up. Here are just a few...

• *The American Journal of Clinical Nutrition* reported a study that showed that fish oil lowers triglyceride levels. Triglycerides are fats in your blood linked to heart disease. The participants took a fish oil supplement or a placebo. Those taking the fish oil had a decrease in triglycerides, which reduced their chance of heart disease by 25%. The subjects taking the placebo showed no significant reduction.

• Cod liver oil helps with depression too. In 1999, the *Archives of General Psychiatry* published an intriguing study that proved a link. Depressed patients took a fish oil supplement or a placebo for 4 months. An overwhelming 64% of patients taking the fish oil reported a significant reduction in symptoms. (Fish oil works on depression by introducing omega-3s to brain cells. The higher the level of omega-3s, the easier it is for the chemical messenger *serotonin* to carry messages from one brain cell to another. This directly affects symptoms of depression.)

- Researchers from the National Eye Institute found that docosahexaenoic acid (DHA) supports the nerves in the retina. <u>DHA is one of the primary ingredients in cod liver oil</u>. Over 4,500 people from the ages of 60 to 80 participated in the National Eye Institute's study. People who supplemented with cod liver oil were <u>50% less likely to develop macular degeneration</u> that those who didn't.

Find Your Best Natural Sources for Omega-3s

You can get your omega-3 fats from several dietary sources. Fortunately, many of these foods taste great. It will be easy for you to transition them into your current diet.

Fish and seafood: These are the foods richest in omega-3 fatty acids. Cold-water, oily fish are best. Add these foods to your diet two to three times a week, and you'll get all of the omegas you need. If you don't like the taste of fish, a fish oil supplement is an alternative. From three to six grams per day is good. I usually recommend my patients take three capsules (or about a tablespoon) with breakfast and three with dinner.

Wild game: If you don't have access to it, you can order wild game now on the Internet. A good alternative to wild game is grass-fed beef. This is as nutritionally close to wild game as you can get in a domesticated animal. You can order it over the Internet or find a specialty farm near you. Make this type of protein a staple of your diet.

Sacha Inchi Oil: I discovered this ancient best plant source of the omega-3 ALA in the mountains of Peru. It's a vegetarian way to enjoy omega-3's benefits. Sacha inchi has a delicious nutty flavor. Take one to two tablespoons of fresh oil daily. Serve it on salads or cooked vegetables.

Nuts: Nuts are some of the most nutritious snacks you can find. Later in the chapter, I'll tell you which one is my favorite… If possible, I prefer the nuts that still have their protective shell on when I buy them. I avoid the nuts in canisters that have added preservatives or sugars. Eat a handful a day for their omega-3 fats.

Leafy green vegetables: Vegetables like kale, spinach and collards are a good addition to any diet. They provide a host of nutrients, along with omega-3s. They are one of the best sources of ALA. So eat green leafy vegetables daily. Steam them to preserve all of their value.

Eggs: Eggs are one of the best sources of good quality omega-3s. Fresh eggs, directly from the chicken are best. But not all of us have that luxury. When you go to the grocery store, look for eggs labeled "cage-free" and "hormone-free."

Avocados: Avocados are a delicious source of omega-3s. They're great on a salad. I also like to add some spices to mashed avocado and eat it as a side dish with dinner. Add an avocado to your plate whenever possible.

Your Government's Experiment with Your Health...

Remember when TV commercials asked you to give up "dangerous" real butter in favor of "Mother Nature friendly" margarine? The ads and packaging promised heart health by replacing animal fats with a new kind of vegetable fat. These high-profit fats became ubiquitous in packaged foods, fast food, and school lunches.

Decades later, health advocates began voicing their objections. Research began to uncover an alarming inflammation, neurological degeneration, and heart disease link to a by-product of artificial fat production we now know as trans fats.

You may not realize it, but trans fats are actually a hundred years old. Back in 1907, Proctor & Gamble was in the candle making business. In those days, candles were made from tallow, which is a form of animal fat.

As tallow became more expensive, they hired a talented German chemist to come up with a substitute. He invented a way to use *hydrogenation* to turn liquid cottonseed oil into a fatty solid.

As electricity became more common, the need for candles dwindled. Not wanting to waste a proprietary product, someone noticed that it shared properties of lard but was very stable at room temperature. So they called it *Crisco* – and a new craze was born.

Made in a factory, trans fats are patentable and dirt cheap. They can dramatically lengthen the shelf life of a packaged product, sometimes for years. And because these unnatural vegetable oils have no cholesterol, they could be sold as "cholesterol free."

With no knowledge of long-term effects, the FDA approved hydrogenated oils for food, and we began an enormous experiment with the public's health. As shocking as it seems, a product originally used as candles made its way into thousands of foods around the world with no long-term testing.

After decades of very widespread use, numerous studies link trans fats to heart attacks, strokes, and cancer to name just a few of its many problems.

Trans fats are proven to increase your LDL (bad) cholesterol. What's worse is that they *decrease* your HDL (good) cholesterol.[4] They also cause inflammation and rob your brain and heart of the real fats you need. They can also make you fat. Very fat...

Ironically, doctors recommended these "low-fat" products for years, thinking they were helping their patients. Dr. Walter Willett, Chairman of the Department of Nutrition at the Harvard School of Public Health had this to say:

"There was a lot of resistance from the scientific community because a lot of people had made their careers telling people to eat margarine [containing trans-fats] instead of butter... When I was a physician in the 1980's, that's what I was telling people to do and unfortunately we were often sending them to their graves prematurely." [5]

How Much Trans Fat are You Eating Every Day?

Your intake of trans fats should be as low as possible. Zero is best. Here's how some of your favorites stack up:

- McDonald's Deluxe Breakfast — 11 grams
- KFC Original Recipe Chicken Dinner — 7 grams
- McDonald's Large French Fries — 6 grams
- Doughnut — 5 grams
- Mrs. Smith's Apple Pie — 4 grams
- Kellogg's Blueberry Eggo Waffle — 2.11 grams

Notice how fast foods are some of the worst offenders? Who ever imagined that breakfast at McDonald's could be so dangerous? Fish and chicken aren't bad on their own. They turn into unhealthy foods when they are fried in hydrogenated vegetable oils.

If you need nutrition in a hurry and are at the mercy of a fast food chain, try Boston Market. The selection there has little trans fats or processed carbs, and there are several high-protein choices. If you must eat at one of the other fast-food chains, here are some tips to follow:

- Choose their leanest red meat
- Choose grilled fish or chicken over fried
- Hold the trans fat containing salad dressing
- Throw the bun in the garbage
- Skip the vegetable oil cooked fries
- Drink water with your meal

Or you can order take-out from a local seafood restaurant or go to the local supermarket. Supermarkets tend not to be that busy at lunchtime and you can pick up a much healthier lunch in about the same time. Build the meal around a good quality source of protein. A typical favorite lunch for me is:

- Fresh sushi or sashimi
- Individual portion of roasted chicken

- One whole, raw tomato

- Quart of milk

- Peach, plum, or berries for dessert

As common as they are, trans fats can be hard for you to identify. Fortunately, a law was passed in 2006 requiring food makers to label foods containing trans fat. But food producers have found many clever ways to disguise the label. What's more, if a food contains less than 1 gram of trans fat, companies are not required to label them.

That may not sound like a problem, but consider this: If a serving of three Oreos contains 0.5 grams of trans fat, Nabisco – the maker of Oreos – doesn't have to put a warning label on the package. As a result, you may think Oreos are "trans fat free." But if you eat nine Oreos, or three servings, you've consumed 1.5 grams of trans fat!

To avoid trans fat, stay away from any product containing shortening, cottonseed oil, corn oil, soy products, and vegetable oils. You could do as I do and try to avoid food with labels in general. (I also eat real butter.)

You'll find trans fats in cookies, cakes, breads, crackers, potato chips, pudding, pies, frozen foods, salad dressing, "butter" flavored popcorn, and French fries. Even so-called "health" foods like granola bars, high fiber cereals and multi-grain snack chips have trans fats. Most "no cholesterol" margarine is still loaded with trans fat.

Eat Whole Foods that Occur Naturally

- Eat naturally occurring food.

- Don't buy low-fat processed foods.

- Stay on the outer aisles of the supermarket. You'll find whole, unprocessed foods on the perimeter of the store.

- Read labels! If products contain high-fructose corn syrup, artificial sweeteners, or partially hydrogenated vegetable oils, avoid them.

New Food	Advertisement's Claim	What the Ad Doesn't Say	Best Choice
Sports Drink	Hydrate, replace electrolytes, provide endurance, and improve sports performance	Contain HFCS, toxic to liver, impedes performance and increases body fat	Water, water, or … water
Energy Bar	Energy boost and quick compact meal	Contain PHVO, high sodium and the worst junk carbs that rob nutrients and energy	Nuts, boiled eggs, fresh fruit, raw veggies
"Diet" Substitute	Weight loss Lower cholesterol	Contains artificial sweeteners linked to many serious health problems	Original food in place of substitute

Grab Hold of Nature's Healthiest Snack

Over the years, I've seen many of my patients ruin their fat loss goals by snacking on the wrong foods. They get hungry between meals and instinctively reach for the potato chips.

I have a healthy and delicious alternative snack. They are full of heart-healthy nutrients and cancer fighting antioxidants. They're also a great source of omega-3s.

When I was a boy, my grandparents had scores of walnut trees. We would spend a week in the fall spreading the walnuts in the sun on straw mats. Once dried, we'd put them in heavy burlap sacks and load them on the back on my granddad's '53 Ford pick-up.

For me, the best part was riding in the back of the truck with the walnuts to the only store in my town. They would sell them there over the winter months, but we always kept plenty for our family. I think my grandma made everything possible from walnuts. She always said they were good for you. I wonder how she knew…

You see, walnuts have a particular kind of omega-3 called alpha-linolenic-acid, (ALA). In fact, walnuts have more ALA than any other nut.

ALA lowers your cholesterol naturally. Both your overall score and your LDL (bad cholesterol) will drop from eating walnuts.[6] ALA is also anti-inflammatory. This alone can reduce joint pain and help prevent heart disease. In addition, ALA naturally lowers your blood pressure.

Walnuts are also high in antioxidants. If you compare them to other nuts, it's not even close. Walnuts also have a flavonoid called ellagic acid. This powerful nutrient is in several types of berries, and we know it inhibits the growth of cancer cells.[7]

If that's not enough for you, walnuts are very high in arginine. Arginine helps make more nitric oxide (NO). This helps your blood vessels to dilate, which increases blood flow. This is great for your heart. (It also helps men get erections and is how Viagra works.)

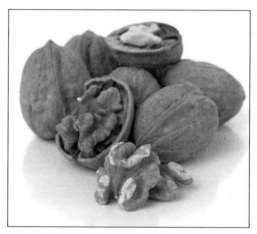

If you're buying walnuts like those we used to sell, in the shell, make sure the shells don't have defects – look for little wormholes. Then, give the nuts a good shake. If they rattle when you shake them, they are probably too old or overdried.

If you prefer unshelled walnuts, look for a freshness date on the package. The high oil content makes them prefer storage in a cool dry place. These essential oils also make them highly perishable. Heat, light and humidity will speed up this process. But store them properly, and they will last for several months.

For walnuts still in their shell, a cool dry storage area will keep them fresh for about six months, up to a year if you put them in the freezer.

Raw shelled walnuts should stay sealed in their original container until you're ready to use them. Their outdate is usually about three to four months. Once you open a package of shelled walnuts, they will last longer if you reseal them and store them in your refrigerator or freezer.

References:

1 Stein R. Low fat diet not disease cure-all. The Palm Beach Post. Feb 8, 2006

2 Stein R. Low fat diet not disease cure-all. The Palm Beach Post. Feb 8, 2006

3 Knopp R. H., et al, "Long-term cholesterol-lowering effects of 4 fat-restricted diets in hypercholesterolemic and combined hyperlipidemic men. The Diet Alternatives Study", Journal of the American Medical Association, Nov 12, 1997; 278(18): 1509-1515

4 Hwang, G, MD, Lee, D, MD, "Trans-fat: The latest and worst fat on the block," Continuing Medical Education, Vol 27, No 2, Feb, 2005:49-54

5 Severson, K, Warner, M, "Fat substitute is pushed out of the kitchen", The New York Times. Feb 13, 2005. p. 23.

6 Feldman EB. The scientific evidence for a beneficial health relationship between walnuts and coronary heart disease. J Nutr. 2002 May; 132:1062S-1101S.

7 Walnuts. WholeHealthMD.com, LLC. 2000

Chapter 8

Step Four – Shift into High Gear with Natural Fat Burners

Now that you've made some important basic changes in the food you eat, let's look at the best supplements to kick your fat loss into high gear. I have used each of these with good success with my patients. They're safe, effective and easy to use.

Back in the old days – before commercial farming – the soil had all the minerals your body needed. Today, chemicals, fertilizers, and overgrowing have depleted the soil, leaving your food with little of the nutrients they used to have. As you'll discover, minerals are essential for achieving and maintaining your ideal weight.

Putting those minerals back into your body will help you burn fat. They will also boost your immune system and help prevent disease.

Before we get to those supplements, I need to address the issue of diet pills. Most of the products you see advertised simply don't work. As we look at the real science of fat loss, you'll see why they won't help you drop those extra pounds.

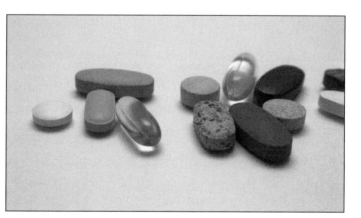

How to Avoid Fat-Loss Frauds

Here's a good example. Go to the website for the diet pill CortiSlim, and you'll see a newly transformed woman saying, *"Stress was piling on the pounds!"* The makers of this diet pill would have you believe that cortisol is to blame. But what *is* cortisol?

Cortisol is your body's main stress hormone. It does a lot more than respond to stress levels. You use it to regulate blood pressure, energy production, immune function, and inflammatory response.

Your cortisol levels are at their lowest when you're healthy and calm. But get stuck in traffic, have a fender bender, or burn your New York strip and cortisol floods into your bloodstream like a dam burst. There's no doubt you release more cortisol during times of stress. *But does cortisol make you fat?*

Popular weight loss products try to link cortisol to weight gain by pointing to the Yale University study published in 2000.[1] It showed that women who respond poorly to stress tend to have more of their fat around the belly. This is the sliver of truth that launched a giant marketing campaign. Excess cortisol could effect where your body stores fat, but it doesn't cause weight gain.

Think about when you've been an overlystressed. When a dog or a caged wild animal is under stress, increased cortisol will cause the dog to lose its appetite. Over time, the dog becomes very thin and starts to waste away. The same is true in humans.

Cortisol suppresses reproduction and long-term management. It gives your body the chance to pool all of its resources to deal with a crisis. Under these conditions, your appetite will disappear. Think back to the last time you panicked or became distressed. Eating was probably the last thing on your mind.

Don't waste your money on these "quick fix" products, hoping that a magic formula will melt away your excess fat. They are empty promises based on incomplete science.

For those who could tolerate the stimulation, ephedra was one of the best. This natural herb was modestly successful at raising your metabolism – but only by a fraction of a percent. This is not enough to make a lasting change in your body. It was banned by the FDA, but that ban was overturned by an appeals court in August 2006. Today, Ephedra is starting to make a comeback.

Ephedra, like the caffeine in your coffee, is a neuro-stimulant. Once inside your bloodstream, your body will down regulate the metabolic process to counter balance the effect of the stimulant. This is why you crave coffee in the morning. You need that jolt to get you back to where you would have been had you not had the coffee in the first place.

One of the more popular fat burners claims that you can eat anything you want and still lose weight. This product uses a less effective Ephedra substitute, synephrine, which is supposed to increase your metabolism without the "harmful stimulants" used in other weight loss products. Also included are caffeine, glucuronolactone, and taurine – the same ingredients found in Red Bull. If you feel any effect, it will be the combination of synephrine and caffeine.

You should think of these as stimulants – not fat burners. They may help wake you up and give you a temporary jolt of energy, but so does a good cup of coffee.

Carb Blockers: Don't Fall for this Diet Deception

Ever since the Atkins Diet hit the market, Americans have been watching their carbs. To ease the guilt that came from eating bagels and pasta, carb blockers seemed like the perfect answer. After all, who wouldn't enjoy French fries knowing that those troublesome carbs conveniently disappear on the way down?

It sounds magical until you realize that carb blockers actually inhibit an important digestive enzyme.

The idea of taking a substance that will interfere with your body's ability to digest food is not a good one. In fact, it's dangerous. Your body absorbs essential vitamins and nutrients in the form of carbohydrates. By blocking them, you are robbing your body of what it needs to survive.

The active ingredient in carb blockers is a white kidney bean extract called *phaseolus vulgaris*. This substance prevents the enzymes in your stomach from digesting starches.

Dietrine, a well-known carb blocker, states on its website that, *"One Dietrine capsule taken prior to a meal can block up to 1125 calories from fat and carbohydrate foods."* Yet there are no reliable clinical studies to support such a claim. In fact, the only reputable study concluded that, in regard to weight loss, *"no statistical significance was reached."* [2]

Worst of all, carb blockers give people a false sense of security. This usually means overeating all of the wrong foods. If you want to lose fat, Nature knows best. Here are a few natural supplements that actually do provide an advantage in burning off extra body fat.

Burn Fat without Exercising or Changing Your Diet

Chromium maintains proper blood sugar by increasing your sensitivity to insulin. It's like instant protection from fat, obesity and diabetes. What's more, chromium supplements can improve glucose tolerance and normalize insulin levels naturally.

On the flip side, people low in chromium suffer from chronically high blood sugar, find themselves packing on the pounds and ultimately can fall victim to diabetes. And having a deficiency of chromium is very common. An estimated 90% of all Americans consume less than the recommended amount of chromium each and every day.

What's more, if you exercise regularly you'll need even larger amounts of chromium than your sedentary neighbors. Active men and women excrete more chromium than couch potatoes do.

Chromium also does wonders for your cholesterol and triglyceride levels. Studies show chromium can lower cholesterol and triglycerides by nearly 20%. Remarkably, chromium can help you burn fat – even if you don't exercise.

About 10 years ago, Dr. Gil Kaats and a team of researchers from the Health and Medical Research Foundation and the University of Texas Health Science Center studied over 150 people to see if they would lose fat just from taking chromium.

They split them into three groups. One group received a placebo (dummy pill). The other two groups received chromium: One got 200 micrograms a day, and the other got 400 micrograms a day.

The participants were told not to change anything about their diet, exercise habits, or how much they ate. In essence, they were allowed to do whatever they wanted.

After three months, the group taking the placebo showed no changes. The 200-microgram group lost an average of 3.4 pounds of body fat. But the 400-microgram group lost an average of 4.6 pounds of body fat – about 35% more. In addition, both chromium groups gained an average of 1.4 pounds of muscle.

Chromium controls your appetite, especially cravings for sweets. It also has the ability to carry protein where your body needs it most. This helps you lose fat while building lean muscle mass.

I've treated hundreds of patients with chromium with good results. When you're looking for a chromium supplement, make sure you take either chromium picolinate or chromium polynicotinate. They're the most effective forms.

The above study used either 200 or 400 microgram doses. I use a 600 microgram chromium picolinate supplement with my patients once a day with food. It's best if you take it with meals.

Magnesium: The Fat Loss Mineral

Like chromium, magnesium quickly boosts your body's response to insulin – exactly what you need to lose fat fast. And not surprisingly, many are deficient of this critical mineral.

Thousands of years ago, your caveman ancestors got plenty of magnesium every day from their native diet – as much as 800 mg to 1,500 mg. But today, you're lucky to get 200 mg. And that's bad news... Magnesium is responsible for over 300 biological and enzymatic functions in your body.

Symptoms of low magnesium are surprisingly similar to what many doctors call metabolic syndrome, or "syndrome x." This chronic disorder increases your risk of each of these:

- Obesity

- Insulin resistance

- High blood pressure

- Low HDL (good cholesterol)

- High triglycerides (blood fat)

- Diabetes

In a recent study published in the *Journal of the American College of Nutrition*, researchers found that simply having enough magnesium in your diet lowers your level of insulin and helps you control your blood sugar.

I've said before that insulin tells your body how much fat to make and store. And keeping your insulin in check is one of the keys to fat loss.

Starchy, high-carb foods spike your blood sugar, triggering insulin. Over time, you become insulin resistant. This puts you on the fast track to obesity, diabetes, and eventually heart disease.

Magnesium helps regulate insulin. But 75% of Americans don't get their recommended daily allowance (RDA) of this vital mineral. And more than 30% don't even get half!

There are several reasons: Commercial farming methods use depleted soil, which makes it almost impossible for your food to soak up magnesium as it grows. And many processed foods have little or no mineral content by the time they end up in the freezer section of your local grocery store.

And magnesium used to be in your drinking water but, water with high mineral content – hard water – fell out of favor because most people don't like the taste.

Think of magnesium as your "fat-loss mineral." Restoring your magnesium levels to that of your caveman ancestors will take you a step closer to your real native diet – the kind you were designed to eat.

You can add magnesium to your diet by eating nuts, seeds, dairy products, and dark green, leafy vegetables. You can also take a supplement. For better absorption, I recommend spending a little extra and getting the chelated form.

In the process of chelation, amino acids form a protective structure around the magnesium ions, helping them pass into the digestive tract where they can be better absorbed. For long-term success, this is the better option.

In most cases, an effective dose is 300 to 400 mg daily. If you have kidney problems or high-degree heart block, don't take any magnesium supplements until you talk to your doctor.

Get Past the Hoodia Hype and Accelerate Your Fat Loss

There's a cactus from southern Africa that has made news as Nature's "diet herb."

It's been featured on *60 Minutes*, the *Today Show*, *ABC News*, and *Oprah*. Many claim it works wonders. Others say it doesn't work at all. I'm talking about Hoodia.

Hoodia comes from the Kalahari Desert in southern Africa. For an estimated 20,000 years, the native Bushmen have used Hoodia to kill their appetite on long hunting trips.

Recently, researchers discovered that the plant has a molecule previously unknown to science. They named it P57. This molecule sends a message to your brain telling you that you're full. The absence of hunger, usually lasting the whole day, means that you can more easily avoid the foods that make you fat. For some, the weight loss is dramatic.

Hoodia was featured on a *CBS News* special report. A team went to remote locations in Africa to see if it really worked. They concluded that Hoodia reduced the desire to eat for an entire day, and unlike most diet pills, Hoodia produced no aftereffects – no upset stomach, no funny taste, no heart palpitations.[3]

Another team from the BBC traveled to the Kalahari for a first hand look with the following story[4]:

"At about 6pm, I ate about half a banana size (piece of hoodia) – and later so did my cameraman. Soon after, we began the four-hour drive back to Capetown. The plant is said to have a feel-good almost aphrodisiac quality, and I have to say, we felt good. But more significantly, we did not even think about food. Our brains really were telling us we were full. It was a magnificent deception. Dinnertime came and went. We reached our hotel at about midnight and went to bed without food. And the next day, neither of us wanted nor ate breakfast. I ate lunch but without appetite and very little pleasure. Partial then full appetite returned slowly after 24 hours."

Hoodia seems to be a dieter's dream. Yet it's unlikely that you will be able to benefit from a Hoodia supplement anytime soon. Drug giant Pfizer was involved in the initial research. They withdrew after deciding that it would not be practical to create a synthetic version of P57.

But the only clinical human trial of Hoodia was promising. In 2001, researchers studied overweight but otherwise healthy people. One group received a P57 extract from Hoodia, and a second group received a placebo.

When comparing to the placebo group, the P57 group had:

• A statistically significant reduction in body fat
• A statistically significant reduction in caloric intake
• No adverse side effects

On average, the P57 group ate about 1,000 calories a day less than those in the control group did. To put that in perspective, the average American man consumes about 2,600 calories a day, a woman about 1,900.

Currently, it's very difficult to get Hoodia out of South Africa. Smuggling and illegal trade is rampant. As a result, dozens of bogus Internet companies have sprung up, claiming to have "the real thing."

But when their products are tested, they usually turn up with no Hoodia at all – or less than a tenth of a percent of the active ingredient. By some estimates, up to 80% of Hoodia products are fraudulent.

I advise you to use caution here. Remember… to lose weight over the long term, boosting your metabolism with exercise is still the most effective strategy by far. PACE® works very well to make that approach more effective.

Get set for your fat-burning PACE® program coming in the next chapter.

References:

1 Elissa S. Epel, PhD, et al., Psychosomatic Medicine, September/October 2000, 62:623-632

2 Udani J, Hardy M, Madsen DC. "Blocking carbohydrate absorption and weight loss: a clinical trial using Phase 2 brand proprietary fractionated white bean extract" Altern Med Rev. 2004 Mar;9(1):63-9

3 Epel, 623-632.

4 Udani J, Hardy M, Madsen DC, 63-9.

Chapter 9

Step Five – Train Your Body that It Doesn't Need Fat

Along with diet and supplementation, high-speed weight loss comes from exercise. But not the kind you may be thinking of… Aerobics, cardio and marathons aren't the best way to keep off the fat. In the end, they encourage your body to store more fat.

My PACE® program is the antidote. It flips a "metabolic switch" in your body, putting you in fat-burning mode for up to 24 hours at a time. It takes as little as 10 minutes and burns fat like nothing you've ever tried.

In this chapter, I'll give you a fat-burning PACE® workout you can do right away. First, I'll give you some of the basics. And I'll show you why the exercise you may be doing is only making it harder for you to drop those extra pounds.

Traditional "Cardio" Makes Keeping the Fat off Tough

Many in the exercise industry will tell you that "cardio" is essential for you to burn off your body fat and get lean. This usually means running or doing other long-duration workouts that pound your body for 45 minutes, an hour or more. But there are several problems with this exercise theory.

For starters, consider the experience of body builders. Many of the very leanest people in this sport (some of the leanest people on the planet in fact) insist that part of their secret to get so lean is, "never do cardio."

My patient, JF, former Mr. USA and world-class bodybuilder, is a staunch advocate of "no cardio." He, like many others in his field, told me that avoiding cardio is the only way to keep your muscle while getting extremely lean.

Science backs him up on this too. A new study shows that the muscles of marathon runners actually shrink. When the muscle biopsies of marathon runners were analyzed, researchers found their muscle fiber size had decreased and atrophied.[1]

This is not to advocate body building, but when someone 280 pounds with the incredibly low body fat of 4% reports that he got that lean while *avoiding* cardio and performing "reps" of exertion lasting two seconds in "sets" lasting less than one minute, it makes you question the relationship between duration of exercise exertion and body fat.

And what about the comparison of native hunters to native farmers? Hunters spend less energy in shorter duration bouts but have nearly universally lower body fat than farmers who spend hours of durational exertion in the fields all day. Many factors could account for this observation. But again, the association of shorter exertion with lower body fat raises interests to investigate.

Don't you have to exercise for at least 15 or 20 minutes before you really kick into fat burning mode? Well, sort of… but there's more to it than that.

The Key to High-Speed Fat Loss is *When* You Burn Fat

Your body can select from several fuel sources. It can burn fat; it can burn carbohydrates like glycogen; or it can get energy from breaking down protein. When you exercise for different durations or at different levels of intensity, it alters the relative proportion of energy you derive from these three sources.

For the first couple of minutes, your body uses something called ATP, the most readily available source of energy. But your supply of ATP is limited. After two to three minutes, your body switches to carbs stored in muscle tissue. This lasts for 15 to 20 minutes before you switch to fat.

As you'll see, this means that your PACE® routines are very short, never lasting for more than 15 to 20 minutes. But your body makes fuel choices based on your activity level as well.

Look at the following table.

What Your Body Burns for Fuel during Various Activities			
Activity Level	Protein	Carbs	Fat
Resting	1 – 5%	35%	60%
Low Intensity	5 – 8%	70%	15%
Moderate Intensity	2 – 5%	40%	55%
High Intensity	2%	95%	3%

Adapted from: McArdle W.D. 1999. Sports & Exercise Nutrition. NY: Lippincott Williams & Wilkins

From reviewing the chart, you see that at low intensity activity your body derives most of its energy from carbohydrates and only 15% from fat. When you look at the lifestyle of our ancient ancestors, this makes sense. Low intensity activity, like walking long distances, was natural for hunter-gatherers.

But when you step up your activity level to moderate, you increase the percentage of the energy burned from fat to 55% of the total. Now notice that if you increase your activity to high intensity you dramatically reduce your dependency on fat and derive nearly all your energy from carbs.

This relationship has led many to advise that you should exercise at moderate intensity because that's how you burn the most fat. Although this seems logical, it turns out to be completely the wrong advice for getting lean.

Spending Endless Hours at the Gym Only to Build More Fat

Burning fat while exercising signals to your body that it needs the fat. This trains your body to make more fat for the next time you exercise. Your body then replenishes your fat each time you eat and becomes efficient at building and preserving fat necessary for long mid-level cardiovascular sessions in preparation for the next endurance workout. In doing so, it sacrifices muscle and other high-energy burning tissues and preserves fat.

So don't bother trying to use this strategy to lose body fat. Your body will fight you in the effort, and you can only do it by sacrificing lean tissue like muscle and internal organs.

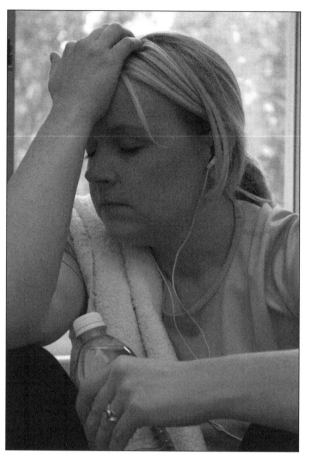

And if the sole purpose of activity is to maximize the proportion of energy derived from fat, why not just rest? Notice from the table that the body burns an even higher percentage of energy as fat (60%) *while resting.* The cardio proponents seem to overlook this fact.

In this way, durational exercise stimulates your body to build fat that it will need to fuel the next episode. Then, if you stop your cardio, you'll put on fat quickly. And many find they have to stop because this unnatural activity has caused degeneration of their joints.

And another point: If you persist through middle age and beyond, it accelerates some very negative effects of aging. It lowers testosterone and growth hormone, boosts destructive cortisol levels, and robs you of muscle, bone, and internal organ mass and strength.

But short duration exercise actually *increases* levels of growth hormone. Researchers from Loughborough University in Leicestershire, England, tested growth hormone levels in sprinters and endurance athletes. On average, the sprinters had three times as much growth hormone as the endurance runners.[2]

But the biggest point that they have missed is this: The most important changes from exercise occur *after, not during,* the exercise period. The way you exercise affects your metabolism for several days.

The important changes begin after you *stop* exercising. This is good news. It means that all you have to do *during* your exercise is to stimulate the adaptive response you need. Then, your body will continue making the important changes afterwards – while you rest.

Kick Start Your Body's Natural Fat Burner

Short bursts of exercise tell your body that storing energy as fat is inefficient, since you never exercise long enough to utilize the fat during each session. Carbohydrates, which are stored in muscle rather than fat, burn energy at high rates. Exercising for short periods will use these carbs and burn much more fat *after* exercising while you replenish the carbs. Short interval exercise creates an "after burn," which can last up to 24 hours after you finish.

Researchers at Laval University in Quebec divided participants into two groups: long-duration and repeated short-duration exercisers.[3] They had the long-duration group cycle 45 minutes without interruption. The short-term interval group cycled in numerous short bursts of 15 - 90 seconds, while resting in between.

The long duration group burned twice as many calories, so you would assume they would burn more fat. However, when the researchers recorded their body composition measurements, the interval group showed that they lost the most fat.

In fact, the interval group lost nine times more fat than the endurance group for every calorie burned. Doesn't this defy the laws of physics? No, it just illustrates that exercise continues to affect your metabolism after you stop. The short bursts stimulated a greater *after burn*.

In addition, short duration bursts produce many other desirable results for your metabolic health:

• Improves maximal cardiac outputs

• Promotes the development of quicker cardiac adjustments to changes in demand

- Helps you lose body fat with as little as 10 minutes per day

- Achieves "higher peak stroke volumes during overload" (Your peak stroke volume is the maximal amount of blood your heart can pump per beat when maximally challenged.)

- Improves cholesterol levels (Subjects in a study of exercise bursts showed a decrease in total cholesterol and an increase in "good" cholesterol.[4])

- Provides an anti-aging benefit by raising testosterone levels, which fights against memory loss, accumulation of fat, low libido, sexual dysfunction, and loss of strength and bone[5]

- Helps you lose weight by burning much more fat after you stop exercising

And you'll be able to get these benefits with much less of your time – no need to spend hours at the gym.

So the recent "cardio craze" was a mistake because it produces an unnatural challenge. It also fails to take into account your body's adaptive responses, like shrinking internal organs, shrinking and weakening muscles, decreasing cardiac reserve capacity, and an increasing dependency on body fat for energy.

Give Yourself the "Caveman Challenge" and Burn Fat on Demand

Our ancestors lived in a world where our food fought back. Predators attacked without notice. They had to run or fight – fast and hard. These short bursts of high-output activity fine tuned our ancient ancestors and kept them fit. We still have the same physiology yet have lost that kind of challenge.

To "reactivate" your native fitness and stay as lean as your ancient ancestors, a few simple techniques will ensure your success.

To burn fat during your PACE® session, create an "oxygen debt." This happens when you ask your lungs for more oxygen than they can provide in that moment. To do it, simply exercise at a pace you can't sustain for more than a short period.

How do you know if you are doing this?

Simple. Monitor your heart rate while you're doing PACE®. When you finish a set, you should see your heart rate go up a few points immediately after you slow down. If you do this successfully, you will feel yourself start to pant.

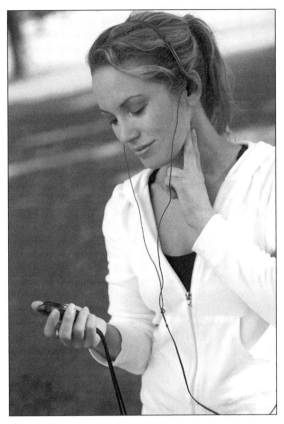

The difference between the oxygen you need and the oxygen you get is your oxygen debt. This will cause you to pant and continue to breathe hard even after you've stopped the exertion until you replace the oxygen you're lacking.

Here's another example: Let's say you pedal as fast as you can on a bike for 15 seconds. When you stop, you continue to pant. This is the kind of high-output challenge you can't sustain for very long. This is very different from doing an aerobic workout for 45 minutes.

By making small changes in the same direction, your workouts can produce remarkable results. And you only need a few minutes to achieve the desired effect.

In a matter of weeks, you can:

• Lose pounds of belly fat
• Build functional new muscle
• Reverse heart disease
• Build energy reserves available on demand
• Strengthen your immune system
• Reverse many of the changes of aging.

PACE® is Your Proven Blueprint for High-Speed Fat Loss

PACE® stands for <u>P</u>rogressively <u>A</u>ccelerating <u>C</u>ardiopulmonary <u>E</u>xertion. The PACE® program starts with interval training, but takes it a step further. Let's look at how these principles are unique to PACE® and how they work together to create a healthy heart and a fat-free body.

Progressivity – Repeated Changes in the Same Direction

Exercise is much more effective when you do a little more of one component each time you do it. <u>Progressivity changes in the same direction</u>. Rather than exercising for longer periods, you increase your intensity levels. As your heart capacity increases, you should add resistance or pick up your pace gradually.

Progressivity is also the need to change your routine over time (more on this later). Doing the same routine over and over, whether cardio or weight training, will lead to failure. Your body needs a consistent set of new challenges in order to grow and achieve.

These changes, made over time, embody the concept of **progressivity**.

Acceleration – Adapting Faster to Demands

As you train your body to respond faster each time you exercise, your physical condition improves. Then, as your body responds more quickly – by increasing your pace, or the resistance, in each progressive workout session, it adapts to the demands. This is the principle of **acceleration.** It is the best way to gear up for unexpected increases in cardiac demands.

When you first begin exercising, it will take several minutes to get your heart rate and breathing up. This is your low cardiopulmonary capacity, or deconditioned phase. But as you begin moving at a faster pace, you'll condition yourself to meet the challenge.

By starting at a comfortable exercise level, you'll enhance your response capacity by increasing your pace sooner in each workout as you progress. The quickness of the demand each time accelerates the development of your adaptive capacity.

This experience tells your body that it needs to increase your lung volume in order to deal with the increased demand for oxygen. It also builds the critical reserve capacity your heart needs to function at its strongest.

Lung volume and reserve capacity are the two key principles of anti-aging. By creating an oxygen deficit after each interval, you are building the body of a warrior. A body that builds muscle and burns fat.

In addition, the oxygen deficit tells your body to burn the glycogen stored in your muscle as fuel. This is essential for fat burning. As you are beginning to see, fat burning happens *after* you finish your workout. Why?

If you burn glycogen (a form of carbohydrate) while you exercise, your body will burn fat after the workout in order to restore its fuel levels in your muscle tissue. If you do this repeatedly, your body becomes used to burning fat after each workout.

PACE® puts your body into fat burning mode – *automatically!*

Start Your High-Speed Fat Loss with this Easy PACE® Routine

If you're new to PACE®, this is a good place to start. You can customize this program to fit your current level of conditioning. Try using a stationary bike or elliptical machine at your local gym. Once you get the feel for it, you can use other machines or run or bike outside.

Have a look at the chart below: The term *level* refers to the resistance. This will make it harder to run or pedal, depending on which machine you start with. The term *RPM* tells you how fast to go.

As you progress, you'll accelerate by going faster (RPM) and boost your intensity by increasing the resistance (level).

Each set has two periods, an *exertion* period and a *recovery* period. During your exertion period, you'll exercise at a level that gives your heart and lungs a challenge. Finding that level will depend on how fit you are.

During your recovery period, you'll relax and let your heart rate slow to your resting rate. Bringing your heart rate down between sets is a key component to PACE®.

Now that you know the basics, let's get started…

Your 20-Minute PACE® Fat Burning Program:

Warm-Up Level 2 50 RPM	Set 1 Level 2 75 RPM		Set 2 Level 5 75 RPM		Set 3 Level 8 125 RPM	
	Exertion	Recovery	Exertion	Recovery	Exertion	Recovery
3 min	2 min	2 min	90 sec	2 min	1 min	2 min

Set 4 Level 10 150 RPM		Set 5 Level 12 185 RPM		Set 6 Level 8 125 RPM		Cool Down Level 2 50 RPM
Exertion	Recovery	Exertion	Recovery	Exertion	Recovery	
30 sec	1 min	30 sec	1 min	1 min	1 min	2 min

Start with a 3-minute warm-up at level 2, pedaling on the stationary bike or running on the elliptical at 50 rpms. This should feel easy and require little effort. After three minutes, start your first exertion period. For the first two minutes, you're going to increase your speed but stay at level 2.

After your first exertion period, begin your first recovery period. During your recovery period, slow down to an easy pace, as if you're walking. You don't need to stop moving during your recovery, but you can if you need to. Simply slow down and go at a slow, easy speed. Focus on normalizing your breathing and tell your mind and body to relax. This gives your body a chance to rest and recover.

In this way, you train your ability to recover from exertion and stress. This also helps your body to burn fat for hours after you finish your routine.

Now that you have a feel for it in your first set, simply repeat the process for your second set. Start your next exertion period and follow it with a recovery period. Each time, increase your speed and intensity. You'll soon get into the groove of exercising in short bursts followed by periods of recovery.

At this stage, you're taking on new ideas and new challenges and giving your body a chance to adapt. And this *adaptive response* is critical for fat loss.

Modern science tends to view your body as a lifeless machine. If something breaks down, simply replace the part and move on. But your body is a living organism with its own sense of timing, intelligence, and connection to its environment. Your body makes decisions based on what you subject it to. It can think, react, and make changes.

The PACE® program works with your body. By giving it the right set of challenges, it enables your body to make adaptive responses that result in weight loss, fat burning, and a buildup of reserve capacity in your heart and lungs.

This gives you the opportunity to transform your body – no matter how overweight or out-of-shape you were when you started. By starting with this simple 20-minute workout and giving your body new challenges over time, you are guaranteed to burn fat like a champion.

Now that you know one of the best ways to burn fat, you are ready to move on to the next chapter to learn how to keep that fat off longer by staying younger.

References:

1 Trappe S, Harber M, et al. Single muscle fiber adaptations with marathon training. J Appl Physiol, 101:721-727, 2006.

2 Van Helder WP. et al., Effect of Anaerobic and Aerobic Exercise of Equal Duration and Work Expenditure on Plasma Growth Hormone Levels, Eur J Appl Physiol 52 (1984) : 255-257.

3 Metabolism 1994; 43: 814-818

4 Medicine and Science in Sports and Exercise 2002; 34: 1468-1474.

5 Kraemer, WJ, et al., Effects of heavy-resistance training on hormonal response patters in younger vs. older men, Journal of Applied Physiology 1999: 87 (3) 982-992.

Chapter 10

Step Six – Stay Leaner Longer by Growing Younger

An effective anti-aging strategy makes your fat loss faster. In fact, it's critical to your long-term success. Consider these points:

- As we age in general, we get fatter. We lose muscle mass every year after age 30. That lost muscle is replaced by fat.

- Overweight people age faster. All the markers we use to measure biological age worsen in overweight people. Fat literally speeds up aging.

- Interestingly hormones control both your aging process and the processes that your body uses to make and store fat. They are the true "task masters" of your body.

Control your hormones and you control how you look, how well you age, and how lean you stay. In this chapter, I'll show you how to safely and naturally alter your endocrine system's production of critical hormones to get leaner faster. At the same time, you'll slow down your aging clock and feel younger longer.

Master the Five Physical Changes of Aging for Long-Lasting Fat Loss

You know that as you get older, you're going to change both physically and chemically. Unfortunately, these biological changes are mostly for the worse. Yet if you effectively address these physical "age markers," your health span will soar, and you'll look and feel younger.

I've measured how physical capacities change with age. Then, I've tracked each change against efforts to reverse them. I'd like you to first focus on the five important *physical* age changes that you can reverse. Then you'll focus on the five *biochemical* changes you can learn to control and change for the better.

1 – Loss of Strength

The first physical marker of aging is muscle. People who age well, who seem to be far younger than their years, are well muscled. This healthy muscle protects your body from aches and pains, disease, and other age related ailments…

Lean Tissues Protect You from Many Age-Related Ailments:
• Reduces Risk of Bone Fractures By Supporting Bones
• Improves Sexual Health By Stimulating Sexual Hormone Production
• Makes You Appear Younger By Stimulating Human Growth Hormone
• Keeps You Trim By Boosting Your Metabolic Rate
• Gives You More Energy By Storing More Glycogen
• Decreases Risk of Disease By Strengthening Your Immune System
• Prevents Chronic Pain By Building Surrounding Tissues and Ligaments

Muscle loss begins at age 30. From then on, you lose an average of three pounds of muscle every decade. Most people feel a bit weaker but for the most part, they don't notice any difference in size. Why? Because this muscle is replaced with *fat*. But it doesn't have to be that way. Muscle loss is preventable and completely *reversible*. I've seen patients of all ages regain *100%* of their youthful muscle mass!

To really make a difference, muscle-building exercise must engage the biggest muscle groups in your body: the quadriceps, the gluteus muscles, and the hamstrings. Perform exercises that flex and extend the hip joint. Practice exercises that *provide resistance through a broad range of motion at the hip joint*. This can include weight training, bicycling, stair-steppers and elliptical machines, or walking up and down stairs. This will boost your metabolism and speed fat loss. (For more on muscle, see chapter 4.)

2 – Increasing Body Fat

Increasing body fat is the second physical marker of aging. If you don't act to prevent it, fat slowly but relentlessly moves into your cells and pads your waist for no reason other than age. But again, this shift is by no means inevitable. You can manage it if you know how.

Several tests can identify and track this change in fat. The most accurate test is the hydrostatic body fat test. It works like this: You get into a tank of water and go under. Test takers record your weight while you're underwater. You can get a hydrostatic test at some health clubs, university health centers, and hospitals. You can also measure fat yourself with a set of calipers. What's a youthful body fat range for a man? 10 to 14%.

So you need to drop a few pounds of fat? Don't jump on the treadmill just yet. Fat loss starts with adequate protein. *Overconsume protein, and minimize everything else.* This is the one piece of advice where I get the most resistance. If you can have some faith and try it, you'll see too how much easier it makes losing weight and achieving a more youthful body.

Finally, you need to perform *effective* fat burning exercise. Short bursts of exercise burn fat best. Short bursts will use energy from carbohydrates stored in muscle rather than from fat. Carbs are capable of burning energy at a much higher rate. You then burn much more fat for energy during the recovery period as you replenish the carbs. Short bursts of exercise are better for your heart and lungs too.

3 – Thinning Bones

Bone density loss is the third physical marker of aging. Just like muscle, you lose bone density every year. In fact, research shows adults lose 1% of bone mass annually. With loss of bone minerals, your bones become lighter, more porous, and weaker – and are at greater risk for fracture.[1]

Unfortunately, ordinary X-rays can't detect bone density loss in its early stages. A bone must lose at least a full quarter of its weight before a standard X-ray can see the problem. Instead, get a bone mineral density test (BMD). The best BMDs test the bones of your lower spine and hip. These areas are at higher risk for fracture as you age.[2]

If your BMD detects trouble, you can increase bone density and strength with weight-bearing exercise such as walking, bicycling, swimming or weight training. Focus on increasing intensity in all of these exercises. As you age, taking calcium will have little effect on this hormone-driven loss of bone density. You can help reverse this process with the only vitamin that is actually a hormone, vitamin D. For maximum anti-aging preservation of bone density, take 400 IU of vitamin D daily.

4 – Shrinking Lungs

As the years pass, your lung volume decreases making lung capacity one of the best markers of physical age. Your doctor can give you a pulmonary function test, (PFT) to check your lung capacity. This test is not invasive or dangerous. I find it very valuable at my Center for Health and Wellness to monitor the benefits of exercise at reversing the loss of lung volume that afflicts so many elders.

I have found that the right physical challenge can reverse this loss of lung volume. For fast results, use a progressive exercise plan like my PACE® program. As we discussed previously, the idea behind PACE® is to advance the intensity of your exercise gradually over time. As simple as this seems, very few people do it. But this is what makes all exercise effective.

5 – Diminishing Heart Capacity

Many people don't realize something's wrong with their heart until it's too late, when they're in the emergency room after a heart attack. Yet the real problem started years earlier. You can measure this gradual loss of heart capacity. It's your fifth physical marker of age.

You can easily gauge your heart with a resting and recovery heart rate. To measure the resting heart rate, locate your pulse. Most people use the wrist. If you can't feel the pulse in your wrist, place the same two fingers just to the side of your Adam's apple, in the soft hollow area at the side of your neck.

Your pulse should have a steady, regular rhythm. Count the number of beats for 15 seconds, then multiply by four to get the beats per minute. See how you rank using the chart below.[3]

Check Your Resting Heart Rate	
Fitness Level	Beats Per Minute (bpm)
Normal Adult	60–100
Well-Conditioned Athletes	40–60

Develop the Heart of a Warrior

Now check your recovery heart rate. It's a good gauge of heart fitness. To start, walk out and get the mail or walk around in your house for a couple of minutes. Then take your pulse. Remember the number; it's your normal activity heart rate.

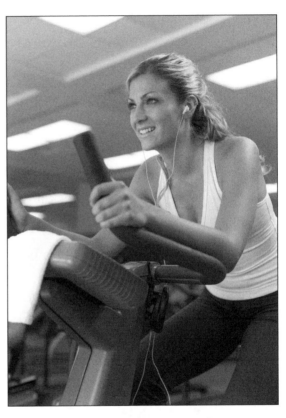

For the next step, begin cardio exercise. Gradually increase the level of intensity in your work effort. Then, at the peak of your intensity measure your heart rate again. Next, decrease your intensity back to normal; then check your heart rate until it's the same as it was when you were walking around. The difference between the peak activity and your normal-activity heart rate is your recovery time. The fitter you are, the faster your heart rate will recover back to normal.

If you don't do much short burst cardiovascular exercise, your cardiovascular system probably needs some work. Here's what to do. When you're performing your PACE® program, exercising with short bursts of exercise, try to get your heart rate within the target range for your age. (These ranges use the maximum heart rate of 220 minus your age.) You can start at 60% of your maximum heart rate. After you've worked with the PACE® program for a few weeks, work up to 80% of your maximum heart rate.

Control these 5 Markers and Maintain Your Ideal Weight for Good

The way your body makes and stores fat has little to do with the saturated fat you'll find in a piece of meat or cheese. The master mechanism is a hormone called insulin. But there are other factors that influence the way you age and gain or lose fat.

If you look in the mirror, you can observe aging as your hair turns gray, your waistline grows, and your body goes soft. But there are biochemical changes underneath that drive this physical aging. Manipulate what happens at the cellular level and you can control the way you age to stay younger longer.

I'm going to show you how to test for and then reverse the chemical bio-markers of aging. Most doctors don't pay much attention to these markers. As you'll discover, this is a BIG mistake if you want to hold onto your youth and slim waistline. I'll show you how to take control of:

- **Insulin** – The overlooked secret to high energy and a lean body.
- **Triglycerides** – More important than cholesterol for heart health.
- **HDL** – The good cholesterol no drug can give you.
- **CoQ10** – The often deficient anti-aging nutrient.
- **Testosterone/Estrogen Ratio** – The key to staying active and ambitious at any age.

Each of these five undergoes a transformation as you age. Taking control of them starts with getting a blood test to check your levels and then using specific anti-aging therapies to improve them. I'm going to share them with you starting with one of the most promising fat loss discoveries ever.

1 – High Insulin is Your Fast-track to Aging and Obesity

When you hear the word "insulin," you think of diabetes. But insulin isn't just about this disease. Even if you aren't diabetic, you can still benefit from having your insulin levels measured. Why? Because insulin plays a key role in aging…

Insulin tells your body to build fat. The more insulin you have, the more fat you'll pack on. Most hormones decline with age, but insulin increases with age. If you want to stay lean, strong, and vigorous at any age, keep your insulin low.

Optimize Your Insulin	
Risky	20 and up
Normal	11 to 20
Best Anti-Aging	4 to 10

To control insulin it's very important you maintain your blood sugar with a low-carb diet. Remember, focus on protein and avoid processed foods. Use the Glycemic Index as a guide to help you choose the healthiest carbs. And remember to exercise.

2 – Don't Miss this Critical Factor for Avoiding Heart Disease

Triglycerides are a type of fat in your blood. High levels put you at risk of heart disease. What's more, as you age, your triglycerides can rise. That's why it's essential to get a triglyceride test. Here's an idea of where yours should be if you want to maintain a healthy heart[4]:

The Truth About Your Triglycerides	
High	200 mg/ dl or higher
Risky	150 to 199 mg/dl
Best Anti-Aging	Less than 100 mg/dl

The most effective way to lower triglycerides is to make the focal point of your diet lean protein. Protein from fish and grass-fed beef is best because these animals have healthy levels of omega-3s. These good fatty acids will also help to reduce your triglycerides, not to mention your waistline.

3 – HDL: The Longevity Lipoprotein

HDL is the good kind of cholesterol. HDL delivers life-giving nutrients and helps remove the bad LDL cholesterol from your arteries. Although a certain amount of LDL in your blood is normal and healthy, excess LDL often accumulates in elders. When this happens, doctors often prescribe cholesterol-lowering drugs.

But if your doctor tries to put you on cholesterol-lowering medication, be warned. Those drugs DO lower LDL, but they don't increase HDL – and that's what matters. Whether you have high cholesterol or not, you should work to increase your HDL to above 80.

The Truth About Your HDL	
Risky	40 or Below
Normal	Between 40 and 80
Best Anti-Aging	Above 80

The best way to increase your HDL is with high intensity, short duration exercise such as my PACE® program that you read about in chapter 9.

4 – Replenish this Nutrient and Forget about Heart Disease – *Forever!*

CoQ10 plays a key role in creating the energy you use to function. It's an antioxidant and can help prevent and even *reverse* heart disease. CoQ10 can improve your immune system, reverse gum disease, and increase your overall energy.

Unfortunately, CoQ10 levels decline with age, as much as 80%. Studies link this decline to the diseases and illnesses of aging, especially cardiovascular problems.[5] In fact, most of my heart patients have turned out to be deficient in CoQ10.

You can measure this critical nutrient in your blood, but very few doctors order the test. You will have to ask. It's imperative you get your levels checked and see how much CoQ10 anti-aging power you're missing. Then you can start doing something about it. First, you can add more CoQ10 to your diet by eating red meat and eggs.

However, modern animal husbandry has led to lower levels of this anti-aging wonder, so supplementation is important. For maximal anti-aging benefit, I recommend taking between 150 to 300 mg per day.

5 – Testosterone: This Vital Force Powers Up Your Fat Loss

We all know that testosterone is the hormone that makes a man a man. But this hormone does much more than that. And it's critical for women too… Testosterone helps to control body fat, mood, energy, sexual desire, cognitive function, and yes, even aging.

> ## The 7 Powers of Testosterone
>
> - Improves Sexual Performance
> - Promotes Libido
> - Stimulates Fat Loss and Muscle Growth
> - Increases Energy Levels
> - Improves Memory, Mood and Mental Clarity
> - Builds Stronger Bones
> - Keeps Urinary and Reproductive Systems Healthy

These are all characteristics of youth. But of course, time begins to work against you, robbing you of vital testosterone as the years pass. Your testosterone levels peak in your twenties, but by age 80, they've dropped between 50% and 70%.[6] And by this time, you've lost muscle, energy, mental clarity, bone density, and sexual ability. Keep your testosterone up, and you slow down the loss of these features that occur with age.

The higher your estrogen, the fatter you'll be. The key here is controlling the ratio between testosterone and estrogen. In our modern world, both men and women have rising levels of estrogen in their blood. And this estrogen excess tips the scales, throwing off the balance between the two.

You can improve your testosterone levels and regain all of the health benefits that go with it from restored libido to better energy and strength. What's more, you don't have to take drugs to do it.

There are a variety of herbal remedies that will gently and naturally raise your testosterone levels and rev up your sex drive. Here are a few I've been using with my patients for decades, with real results:

- **Horny Goat Weed** This is an aphrodisiac first used in China over a thousand years ago. Interestingly, it improves blood flow by increasing levels of nitric oxide (NO), which is exactly how Viagra works. In women, it stimulates the blood flow needed during sexual arousal. It also acts on the neurotransmitters in the brain that stimulate sexual response.

- **Terrestris Tribulus** Discovered by the ancient Greeks, this powerful herb boosts both libido and testosterone levels. Decades of clinical research have proven its effectiveness.[7] It also increases muscle strength and acts as a powerful antioxidant.

- **Avena Sativa** This herb boosts "free" testosterone levels in the blood. Almost all of the testosterone in your body is "bound" to proteins that direct it towards tissue growth and other physiological processes. Only about 2 percent of testosterone is "bio-available." It's free testosterone that will really get you humming. And Avena Sativa gives you more of it.

Bringing your estrogen down is just as easy. There's a natural compound called **DIM**, which metabolizes excess estrogen and flushes it from your blood stream. It's a concentrated form of what you find in cruciferous vegetables like broccoli and cauliflower.

I've used DIM with patients for years. It's safe and very effective. You can find it, along with the testosterone boosters mentioned above, at your local health food store or vitamin shop. And be sure to let your doctor know you're taking them.

Now on to Step Seven.

References:

1 Frank, Bill. Forever Young: 100 Age-Erasing Techniques, New York, NY: HarperCollins, 2003, p. 94-98.

2 Bone Mineral Density Test Overview, WebMd in collaboration with Healthwise, Incorporated, August 2004. http://my.webmd.com/hw/osteoporosis/hw3738.asp?lastselectedguid={5FE84E90-BC77-4056A91C-9531713CA348

3 Pulse Measurement Test Overview. WebMd in collaboration with Healthwise, Incorporated, August 2004. http://my.webmd.com/hw/heart_disease/hw233473.asp?lastselectedguid={5FE84E90-BC77-4056-A91C-9531713CA348}

4 High Triglycerides.WebMD in collaboration with HealthWise Incorporated, August 2004 http://my.webmd.com/hw/heart_disease/zp3388.asp?lastselectedguid={5FE84E90-BC77-4056-A91C-9531713CA348}

5 Report of the Expert Committee on the Diagnosis and Classification of Diabetes Mellitus. Diabetes Care 20(7) 1997, 1183*1197.

6 Wright J. Maximize Your Vitality and Potency, Smart Publications, CA: 1999

7 Gautham K, et al, "Aphrodisiac properties of Tribulus Terrestris extract," Life Sciences, 2002 9;71(12):1385-96.

Chapter 11

Step Seven – Enjoy Your Success the Easy Way

You now have everything you need to kick-start your own high-speed fat loss program. Many times, after I've given these effective fat loss tools to patients, they respond with, *"Sounds great, Doc… but how do I get started?"*

It's not as hard as you might think. Here is your core game plan.

First, remember this basic formula to keep you on the right track:

High Protein + Low Carbs + Good Fats + PACE® = High-Speed Fat Loss

Make it your new mantra. Learn it, know it, live it. Every food you choose – and every exercise you do – should follow this guideline.

This simple advice will bring you in line with your **native diet**. This is the diet that kept your ancient ancestors strong, lean, and full of strength. Back in those days, they ate only what they could hunt and gather. Everything was fresh and full of nutrients. And they never ate grains or sugar.

Over the course of 2.5 million years, the human body evolved on a diet of meat, fruit, seeds, nuts, and vegetables. In fact, human survival became genetically dependent on these foods.

Your genetic makeup is 99.995% identical to that of your caveman relatives. But your diet has changed drastically. Over 70% of your diet was not available to your ancient ancestors.

That means you're not eating the foods your body needs… the foods that you were born to eat. All those grains, sugars, and processed foods were never part of Nature's plan for you. And our addiction to them is at the core of the chronic disease epidemic that takes the lives of millions of Americans every year.

How to Choose High-Speed Fat Loss Foods

Protein should be the focal point of each meal – especially breakfast. These days, most people reach for bread, doughnuts, and cereals when they get up in the morning. But to drop fat and keep it off, go for high-protein breakfast foods like eggs and meat. Your grandparents' generation had it right when they ate steak and eggs every morning.

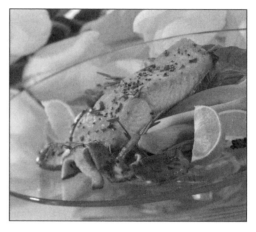

Use this approach for lunch and dinner, too. If not meat, then go for fish or poultry. Extra protein will ensure a metabolic shift towards fat burning. To speed the process, get another shot of protein from supplements. ***Whey protein isolate*** powder will help you burn fat faster. And its effect will not diminish over time. You could take it everyday for the rest of your life and still get all the fat-burning benefits. An extra 25 to 50 mg a day will work wonders.

If you can, eat your eggs raw. I often make a protein shake in the morning and blend in a few raw eggs. As you know, eggs are a perfect source of protein. And their nutrients have more power when you eat them raw. The amino acids that make up the protein go right to work when they're consumed in their raw state. This is exactly what you need for fast energy in the morning.

Your next step is to look at the glycemic index. To help you choose *specific* carbohydrate sources, you'll refer back to this as a guide. Go through each food group and choose three or four low-glycemic foods that you really like. Combine these with your choice of protein at each meal.

Here's an example: For dinner, you have a spinach salad with crushed walnuts, with an olive oil and balsamic vinegar dressing. For your entrée, you have a New York strip steak (grass-fed, only) with a side of sautéed asparagus tips. For dessert, have a sliced peach with plain yogurt and berries. Everything in this meal has a glycemic index less than 40.

With this meal, you also have a good high-quality protein source, some greens, nuts, berries, and omega-3 fats.

Because these foods are all very low-glycemic, they won't direct your body to make as much fat. And when you put this approach to eating with your PACE® exercise program, you'll ignite your fat burning in short order.

Every week or so, go back to your glycemic index and make some new choices. Add these to the mix for variety. If you think of something that's not on the list, go to www.glycemicindex.com and look it up.

You'll get the hang of it quickly. Your native diet is very intuitive, and it's not hard to plan delicious meals once you know the game plan. After a few weeks, you'll stop craving sweets and grains. And you'll have twice the energy.

Accelerate Your Fat Loss by Using Supplements Wisely

Now you should review the supplements in chapter 8. Choose the supplements that make the most sense for you. But remember, they only work long-term if you use them in the context of a balanced, native diet. If you're planning to eat lots of starchy foods, hoping the supplements will "compensate," you'll be disappointed.

Now, let's review the 7 steps to your high-speed fat loss.

A 7 Step Review

1. **<u>Power up your metabolism with protein</u>**.
   Quality protein is your single most important nutritional concern. It is a critical component of every cell in your body. The most important thing to remember is that overconsuming protein is one of the easiest and most reliable ways put your body in fat-burning mode. And choose animal protein because it is the most powerful and more nutritious (grass-fed and cage free).

2. **Test your carbs**.

Keep in mind that when you're considering which carbs to avoid, it's not about sugar or sweetness… It's about "starchiness." Use the glycemic index as your guide. You'll see that starches have the highest scores. They spike your blood sugar the highest and for the longest time.

When your blood sugar rises, it triggers a release of the hormone insulin. And too much insulin makes you fat. For high-speed fat loss choose foods that have a glycemic index below 40 until you get as lean as you want to be. Once you've achieved your goal you can gradually liberalize your glycemic intake. Adding fruit back is usually the best place to start allowing yourself more choices.

3. **Eat the right fats to burn fat**.

Don't forget that not all fats are the same. There are good, bad, and ugly fats. The good fats are the omega-3s that help burn fat. The best sources of omega-3s are grass-fed beef, wild salmon, avocado, walnuts, olive oil, and sacha inchi oil.

The bad fats are the omega-6s. Although you need them for a balanced diet, you only need a modest amount. To avoid getting too much, stay away from things like grain-fed beef, processed foods, and vegetable oil.

The ugly fats are the trans fats. You want to avoid these completely. Try to eliminate all the processed packaged foods like potato chips, cookies, cakes and bottled salad dressings from your diet.

4. **Shift into high gear with natural fat burners**.

Beware of all the fat-loss frauds out there. Avoid diet pills that are nothing more than stimulants and carb-blockers that are dangerous to your health. Instead, opt for the natural fat burners like chromium and magnesium.

5. **Train your body it doesn't need fat**.

The key to remember here is that you don't want to do long duration exercises like aerobics or running marathons because they encourage your body to store fat.

What you want to do are short bursts of exercise that tell your body that storing energy as fat is inefficient, since you never exercise long enough to utilize the fat during each session. PACE® flips a "metabolic switch" in your body, putting you in fat-burning mode for up to 24 hours at a time. It takes as little as 10 minutes and burns fat like nothing you've ever tried.

6. **<u>Stay leaner longer by growing younger</u>**.
This is a great part of the program: An effective anti-aging strategy makes your fat loss easier, faster and more sustainable. Pay special attention to the five physical markers of aging… loss of strength, increasing body fat, thinning bones, shrinking lungs, and diminishing heart capacity. Control these five markers and you will be able to maintain your ideal body fat for good.

7. **<u>Enjoy your success the easy way</u>**.
Remember and live by my easy formula for high-speed fat loss to keep you on track.

High Protein + Low Carbs + Good Fats + PACE® = High-Speed Fat Loss

You're Ready for Success

The way you approach success will have a big impact on your weight loss.

Henry Ford once said, "*Whether you think you can or think you can't, you're right.*" My experience with patients teaches me that you have to believe you will succeed in order to succeed. If you believe you will fail, then you will. So make the conscious note now, decide with intent, and say to yourself: **"I believe in myself!"** Repeat this to yourself daily.

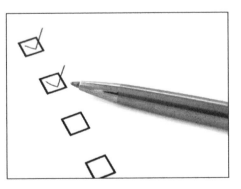

Set goals. Write them down. And, try to be specific as possible. When you write them down you make a commitment to work toward them. You can look at your goals every day to reinforce what it is that you're working toward.

It also helps to track your progress so you can acknowledge your success and recognize that you are taking the necessary steps toward a healthy life. I have provided you with some charts in the next chapter to help you do this.

You now have the tools you need for your high-speed fat loss plan. There's no time like the present to start getting leaner and healthier.

To your good health, always!

Chapter 12

Charts, Guides, and Resources

On the following pages you'll find charts and forms to use to track your progress with your new high-speed fat loss plan. You can either fill out the forms here in the book or copy them to take with you at any time.

Included are the following:

- Pre-Evaluation Form
- Body Composition Chart for Men
- Body Composition Chart for Women
- Circumference Measurements Chart
- PACE® 20 Minute Workout Chart
- Daily Workout Journal
- Meal/Glycemic Log
- Weekly Progress Report
- Final Review
- Resources

I have also included forms for you to write in to me. Let me hear from you on how you are doing. We may be able to use your success in future publications to help others achieve their fat loss goals.

Date	Weight	Chest	Abdomen	Thigh	Sum of Skin Folds	% of Fat	Lbs of Fat	Lean Body Mass

BODY COMPOSITION CHART – MEN

Date	Weight	Iliac Crest (Just Above Hip)	Triceps	Thigh	Sum of Skin Folds	% of Fat	Lbs of Fat	Lean Body Mass
BODY COMPOSITION CHART – WOMEN								

CIRCUMFERENCE MEASUREMENTS (Inches or Centimeters)		
Date	Waist	Hips

PACE® 20 Minute Workout

	Warm Up	Set 1 Level 2 75 RPM		Set 2 Level 5 75 RPM		Set 3 Level 8 125 RPM	
Week		Exertion	Recovery	Exertion	Recovery	Exertion	Recovery
1							
2							
3							
4							

		Set 4 Level 10 150 RPM		Set 5 Level 12 185 RPM		Set 6 Level 8 125 RPM	
Week		Exertion	Recovery	Exertion	Recovery	Exertion	Recovery
1							
2							
3							
4							

	Warm Up	Set 1		Set 2		Set 3	
Week		Exertion	Recovery	Exertion	Recovery	Exertion	Recovery
1							
2							
3							
4							

		Set 4		Set 5		Set 6	
Week		Exertion	Recovery	Exertion	Recovery	Exertion	Recovery
1							
2							
3							
4							

	Warm Up	Set 1		Set 2		Set 3	
Week		Exertion	Recovery	Exertion	Recovery	Exertion	Recovery
1							
2							
3							
4							

		Set 4		Set 5		Set 6	
Week		Exertion	Recovery	Exertion	Recovery	Exertion	Recovery
1							
2							
3							
4							

	Warm Up	Set 1		Set 2		Set 3	
Week		Exertion	Recovery	Exertion	Recovery	Exertion	Recovery
1							
2							
3							
4							

		Set 4		Set 5		Set 6	
Week		Exertion	Recovery	Exertion	Recovery	Exertion	Recovery
1							
2							
3							
4							

Pre-Evaluation

Health and Weight Loss Goals for the Next 10 Weeks: _____
_____
_____

Nutrition Goals for the Next 10 Weeks: _____
_____
_____

Expected or Desired Outcome: _____
_____
_____

Obstacles I May Face in Reaching My Goal: _____
_____
_____

How I Plan on Breaking Through These Obstacles: _____
_____
_____

My Motivation in Reaching My Goals: _____
_____
_____

How I Expect to Feel Once I've Achieved My Goal: _____
_____
_____

Before Picture:

Daily Workout Journal

Date: _____

Today's Goal: _____

Type of Workout: _____

Warm Up	Set 1		Set 2		Set 3	
	Exertion	Recovery	Exertion	Recovery	Exertion	Recovery

Set 4		Set 5		Set 6		Cool Down
Exertion	Recovery	Exertion	Recovery	Exertion	Recovery	Exertion

HEART RATE – RESTING	
TARGET HEART RANGE	ACTUAL RATE

HEART RATE – ACTIVE	
TARGET HEART RANGE	ACTUAL RATE

How I'd Rate My Progress Today: _____

_____

_____

Daily Comments: _____

_____

_____

Meal and Glycemic Log

MEAL LOG		SUPPLEMENTS
Breakfast		
Lunch		
Afternoon Snack		
Dinner		
Evening Snack		

Highest Glycemic Index of Food Today: _____

_____

Glycemic Goal: _____

_____

My GI Score	
CATEGORY	DAILY SCORE
BAKED GOODS	
CEREAL	
BEVERAGES	
DAIRY	
POTATO	
PASTA	
GRAIN	
MEAT	
FRUITS	
LEGUMES	
NUTS	
VEGGIES	
SOUPS	
CANDY	

How Many Different Foods in Each Category Did You Eat? _____

_____

Daily Comments: _____

_____

Meal and Glycemic Log

MEAL LOG		SUPPLEMENTS
Breakfast		
Lunch		
Afternoon Snack		
Dinner		
Evening Snack		

Highest Glycemic Index of Food Today: _____

_____

Glycemic Goal: _____

_____

My GI Score	
CATEGORY	DAILY SCORE
BAKED GOODS	
CEREAL	
BEVERAGES	
DAIRY	
POTATO	
PASTA	
GRAIN	
MEAT	
FRUITS	
LEGUMES	
NUTS	
VEGGIES	
SOUPS	
CANDY	

How Many Different Foods in Each Category Did You Eat? _____

_____

Daily Comments: _____

_____

Weekly Progress Report

Week Ending Stats: _______________

MALE:

DATE	
WEIGHT	
SKIN FOLD MEASUREMENTS	
CHEST	
ABDOMEN	
THIGH	
TOTAL OF SKIN FOLD	
% OF FAT	
LBS OF FAT	
LEAN BODY MASS	

FEMALE:

DATE	
WEIGHT	
SKIN FOLD MEASUREMENTS	
TRICEP	
HIP	
THIGH	
TOTAL OF SKIN FOLD	
% OF FAT	
LBS OF FAT	
LEAN BODY MASS	

Things That Helped My Progress: ______________________________

____

Things That Hindered My Progress: ______________________________

____

Ideas to Keep This From Happening Again: ______________________________

____

Goals Achieved: ______________________________

____

What I'd Like to Accomplish Next Week: ______________________________

____

How I'd Rate My Overall Progress This Week: ______________________________

____

Additional Comments: ______________________________

____

____

____

Weekly Progress Report

Week Ending Stats: _____

MALE:

		FEMALE:		
DATE		DATE	
WEIGHT		WEIGHT	
SKIN FOLD MEASUREMENTS		SKIN FOLD MEASUREMENTS	
CHEST		TRICEP	
ABDOMEN		HIP	
THIGH		THIGH	
TOTAL OF SKIN FOLD		TOTAL OF SKIN FOLD	
% OF FAT		% OF FAT	
LBS OF FAT		LBS OF FAT	
LEAN BODY MASS		LEAN BODY MASS	

Things That Helped My Progress: _____

_____

Things That Hindered My Progress: _____

_____

Ideas to Keep This From Happening Again: _____

_____

Goals Achieved: _____

_____

What I'd Like to Accomplish Next Week: _____

_____

How I'd Rate My Overall Progress This Week: _____

_____

Additional Comments: _____

_____

_____

_____

Final Review

After Picture:

Goals Achieved: _____
_____
_____

What Was My Biggest Success?: _____
_____
_____

What I Did That Worked Well In Helping Me To Achieve My Goals: _____
_____
_____

Things I Could Have Done To Be More Successful: _____
_____
_____

How I'd Like To Maintain/Further My Weight Loss Achievements In The Future: _____
_____
_____

How I Feel Now That I've Achieved My Goal: _____
_____
_____
_____
_____

May we use your success story?

If you'd like to share your story with us and others, please fill out the following two forms (testimonial authorization and photo release) and send them to us at the address below with your before and after pictures, your starting and ending body composition ratings. And tell us about your success story.

Al Sears MD
Attn: Wellness Research and Consulting
12794 W. Forest Hill Blvd. Ste. 16
Wellington, FL 33414

Wellness Research & Consulting, Inc.
Photo Release

I, _____, give Al Sears, MD and Wellness Research & Consulting, Inc. permission to publish taken photo's for promotional, educational and informative materials both online and in print.

_____   _____
Name   Date

_____   _____
Witness   Date

Wellness Research & Consulting, Inc.
Testimonial Authorization

We appreciate your sharing your experience with Wellness Research and Consulting. Please write down your testimonial in the space provided and sign for approval, authorizing Wellness Research and Consulting to use your testimonial in our marketing efforts. Your name and address will be changed to protect your identity.

_____

_____

_____

_____

_____

_____

_____

_____

_____

_____

_____   _____
Print Full Name   Signature

_____
Address

_____
(Area Code) Phone Number

Resources

Wellness Research Foundation - http://wellnessresearch.org/

Life Extension Foundation – http://www.lef.com/

Vitamin Research News – http://www.vrp.com/

News Target – http://www.newstarget.com/

Whole Fitness – http://www.wholefitness.com/

Glycemic Index - http://www.glycemicindex.com/

U.S. Wellness Meats - http://www.grasslandbeef.com/index.html

Alaskan Harvest Seafood - http://www.alaskaharvest.com/

Delicious Organics - http://www.deliciousorganics.com/

World's Healthiest Foods – http://www.whfoods.com/

Eat Wild – http://www.eatwild.com

Stevia Webstie – http://www.stevia.com

Sears, A. *Rediscover Your Native Fitness*, PACE, Wellness Research & Consulting Inc., 2006

Sears, A. *The Doctor's Heart Cure*, Dragon Door Publications, 2004

Robinson, J. *Why Grassfed is Best*, Vashon Island Press: WA 2000

Frank, B. *Forever Young: 100 Age-Erasing Techniques*, HarperCollins, NY, 2003

Schlosser, E. *Fast Food Nation: The dark side of the all-American meal.* HarperCollins, NY, 2001.

Wright J. *Maximize Your Vitality and Potency*, Smart Publications, CA: 1999

Bowden, J. *The 150 Healthiest Foods on Earth*, Fairwinds Press, 2007

Jonny Bowden's website: http://www.jonnybowden.com

Mercola, J. The No-Grain Diet, NY: Penguin Group U.S.A., 2003

Personal Journal

Personal Journal

_____

_____

_____

_____

_____

_____

_____

_____

_____

_____

_____

_____

_____

_____

_____

Personal Journal

Personal Journal

Personal Journal

Personal Journal

_____

_____

_____

_____

_____

_____

_____

_____

_____

_____

_____

_____

_____

_____

Personal Journal

Personal Journal

Personal Journal

Personal Journal

_____

_____

_____

_____

_____

_____

_____

_____

_____

_____

_____

_____

_____

_____

Personal Journal

Personal Journal

Personal Journal

Personal Journal

_____

_____

_____

_____

_____

_____

_____

_____

_____

_____

_____

_____

_____

Personal Journal

Personal Journal

Personal Journal

Personal Journal

_____

_____

_____

_____

_____

_____

_____

_____

_____

_____

_____

_____

_____

_____

Personal Journal

Personal Journal

_____

_____

_____

_____

_____

_____

_____

_____

_____

_____

_____

_____

_____

_____

Personal Journal

Personal Journal

_____

_____

_____

_____

_____

_____

_____

_____

_____

_____

_____

_____

_____

Personal Journal

Personal Journal

_____

_____

_____

_____

_____

_____

_____

_____

_____

_____

_____

_____

_____

_____

Personal Journal

Personal Journal

_____

_____

_____

_____

_____

_____

_____

_____

_____

_____

_____

_____

_____

_____

Personal Journal

Personal Journal

_____

_____

_____

_____

_____

_____

_____

_____

_____

_____

_____

_____

_____

_____

_____

Personal Journal

Personal Journal

Personal Journal

Personal Journal

_____

_____

_____

_____

_____

_____

_____

_____

_____

_____

_____

_____

_____

Personal Journal

Personal Journal

Personal Journal

Personal Journal